PHARMED

The Thief Comes Only to Steal, Kill, and Destroy...

S R Arnold

Book Two of the Trilogy

Some quotations have been lightly adapted for clarity while preserving the meaning of the original text.

Published by S R Arnold

ISBN: 979-8-9956963-1-5

Library of Congress Control Number: 2026911700

Printed in the United States of America

Table of Contents

Introduction: The Pen

You already know something is wrong

You have known it for a while. It is not a single thing you can point to — it is a pattern, a texture, a persistent sense that the world being described to you by the institutions you were raised to trust does not match the world you actually inhabit. The food that is supposed to nourish you leaves you chronically unwell. The medicine that is supposed to heal you manages your symptoms indefinitely without resolving them. The news that is supposed to inform you leaves you more confused and more afraid than you were before you encountered it. The agencies built to protect you seem, on close examination, to be protecting something else.

You have probably said this out loud to someone. You have probably watched their face close.

That closing — that refusal to look, that retreat into the comfort of the official account — is one of the most painful things a person who has seen something clearly can experience. It is the specific loneliness of the awake. You are not speaking from paranoia or from ideology. You are speaking from observation. And the observation is being returned to you labeled as something dangerous to hold.

This book is for you.

It is also for the person who handed it to you — the one who has been trying to tell you something and has not been able to find the words, or the evidence, or the frame that would make you stay in the room long enough to hear it.

And it is for the person who is not yet sure. The one who suspects but has not confirmed, who senses the pattern but cannot yet name it. The skeptic is welcome here. This book will not ask you to trust it. It will ask you to look at what it puts in front of you and evaluate it for yourself. Every significant claim in these pages traces to a primary source: a congressional record, a government investigation, a court document, a peer-reviewed study, the published statements of the principals themselves. You can verify everything. You should.

Let me tell you where this book comes from.

In February of 2020, I was sick for weeks. I did not go to the doctor. I did not know then what I likely had — the world had not yet assembled its vocabulary for what was beginning. I knew I was sick in a way that felt different from anything before, and I knew, with the specific alertness of someone who had been watching the institutional landscape for a long time, that something was wrong with what I was being told about it.

I watched what followed.

I watched a global population told to stay inside, told that the ordinary human need for contact and presence was now dangerous, told that the neighbor who had not complied was a threat. I watched the vocabulary of compliance constructed in real time — the phrases that ended conversations, the labels that disqualified dissent, the mechanisms by which credentialed scientists and physicians who raised legitimate questions found themselves deplatformed, defunded, and professionally destroyed.

I watched people I loved accept injections from a technology that had never before been deployed in human beings at scale, authorized through an emergency framework that explicitly bypassed the long-term safety evaluation that a century of pharmaceutical development had established as the minimum requirement for trust. I watched them get sick. Some recovered. Some did not. Some are chronically ill in ways they cannot explain and that the system refuses to investigate with urgency.

Some of them have died.

I am not the only person who has watched this. You may have watched the same thing in your own family, your own community. The specific grief of it — the watching, the warning that was not heard, the loss that followed, the inability to say plainly what you believe happened because the saying of it places you outside the circle of acceptable opinion — that grief is one of the forces behind this book.

But grief is not the book's purpose. Documentation is.

Because here is what I have come to understand in the years of watching and warning: the people who cannot hear what happened in 2020 cannot hear it not because they are foolish or corrupt but because they have no framework for it. The Covid period did not arrive from nowhere. It was the demonstration — the deployment, at global scale, of an apparatus that had been under construction for a hundred years. If you do not know the apparatus exists, the demonstration looks like a crisis poorly managed. If you know the apparatus, the demonstration looks like exactly what it was.

This book documents the apparatus.

It begins where the apparatus began — not in 2020, not with the names that dominate the current headlines, but with an idea funded by Carnegie and Rockefeller in 1904 that some human beings are raw material. It follows that idea as it became law, as it was imported and refined, as it captured the institutions built to resist it, as it reached into the food supply and the medical system and the regulatory framework and the childhood health infrastructure and the enforcement network that kept the compliant rewarded and the resistant neutralized.

It arrives at 2020 with the full weight of a hundred years of documented institutional history behind it. By the time this book reaches the pandemic period, the reader who has followed the build will not be surprised by what they find. They will recognize it.

And recognition — the moment when the pattern becomes visible and cannot be unseen — is where the real work of this book begins.

The recognition is not comfortable. What the documented record shows is not the product of ordinary institutional failure, ordinary corruption, ordinary greed. Those things explain the individual crime. They do not explain the consistency, the coordination, the century-long patience of the assault, the specific concentration on the human body and human cognition above every other dimension of human life that institutional power could more easily have targeted.

What explains it is what Jesus named plainly in John 10:10:

The thief comes only to steal and kill and destroy.

The men and women who built this apparatus did not originate it. They served it. They sold themselves to the evil one for the things he offered them — wealth, power, protection, the intoxicating certainty of being on the winning side. Many others who participated at lower levels are victims of their own ordinary human weakness — people who wanted security and found that the system rewarded compliance and punished resistance. That is not innocence. Whether or not it is ignorance is not for the author to judge.

This book documents what the theft looked like. What was stolen. From whom. Through which institutions. Over how long. The evidence is in the congressional record, in FOIA-released documents, in the findings of government investigations, in peer-reviewed scientific literature. It does not require you to trust the author. It requires only the willingness to look.

And the same verse that names the thief names the answer to him.

I came that they may have life, and have it abundantly.

That is the rope. It has been in the room since the first sentence.

The one who spoke those words is the one holding the other end, and he has been holding it through everything this book documents — through every program, every capture, every stolen life — without letting go. The final chapters of this book will name the call he has extended and extend it again. It is the oldest call in the world and the only one adequate to what the evidence in these pages demands.

For now: the evidence. All of it. Documented, sourced, verifiable.

This is what was done.

This is what it was done with.

This is who did it.

And this is the one who names it, who warned us it was coming, and who holds the only hope that survives it.

Take heed that no one deceives you.

— Matthew 24:4

The first thing he said.

A note on sources: Every significant claim in this book traces to a primary source — congressional testimony, government investigations, FOIA-released documents, peer-reviewed scientific literature, court records, or the published statements of the principals themselves. Where evidence is contested, that is said plainly. Where a conclusion goes beyond what the documentation supports, that line is marked. The reader is invited — encouraged — to verify independently. The sources are cited with enough specificity that you can find them. In many cases you can find them at home, in minutes. Do not take this on faith. Look.

Chapter 1: The Ideological Root

Galton, Eugenics, Carnegie, Rockefeller, and the Idea That Some Bodies Are Raw Material

"So God created man in his own image, in the image of God he created him; male and female he created them."

— Genesis 1:27

Every assault has an origin. Not always a moment — sometimes an idea, funded by the people with the most to gain from its conclusions, institutionalized across generations until it no longer needed defending because it had become the operating assumption of the systems that governed ordinary life.

The idea that made the century of programs this book documents possible was formulated in 1863 by Sir Francis Galton, a cousin of Charles Darwin, in papers and lectures that culminated in his 1869 book *Hereditary Genius*. The idea was simple: that human beings differ in heritable quality, that those differences can be measured, and that society should manage reproduction to produce more of the desirable and fewer of the undesirable.

Galton called this project eugenics — from the Greek for "well born."

The verse above is placed here not as decoration. It is placed as the document the eugenics movement was explicitly working against. Galton's framework required the rejection of what Genesis 1:27 states: that every human being, without exception of heritable quality, bears the image of God. The eugenics movement did not dispute this verse on theological grounds. It simply proceeded as though the verse were false — as though some human beings were raw material to be managed in the service of institutional goals, and others were not.

That is the idea this book opens with. Because everything that follows was built on it.

I. THE MONEY BEHIND THE IDEA

An idea requires money to become an institution. The American eugenics movement received its institutional foundation from three sources: the Carnegie Institution of Washington, the Rockefeller Foundation, and the Harriman railroad fortune. This is not an allegation from critics of those institutions. It is documented in the institutions' own records, in the published history of the Eugenics Record Office, and in the comprehensive scholarly histories of the movement.

In 1904, the Carnegie Institution funded the Station for Experimental Evolution at Cold Spring Harbor, Long Island — the facility that would become the institutional center of American eugenics research. In 1910, biologist Charles Davenport, armed with a letter of personal endorsement from Galton himself and backed by a grant from Mary Harriman, widow of the railroad baron E.H. Harriman, established the Eugenics Record Office on the same campus. The Carnegie Institution began directly funding the ERO in 1917 and continued as its primary funder until the office closed in 1939. The Rockefeller Foundation provided additional funding throughout.

The ERO's function was to compile pedigree records on hundreds of thousands of Americans, train field workers to gather data from institutions housing the poor, the mentally ill, and the imprisoned, and produce legislative blueprints for what it called "race betterment." Between 1910 and 1924, it trained 258 field workers — most holding bachelor's degrees in biology — to systematically document what it classified as hereditary defects in the American population.

Notice the populations they concentrated on. Not the families of the Carnegie and Rockefeller philanthropists who funded the work. The populations in state institutions, mental hospitals, and prisons — people selected, as the Advisory Committee on Human Radiation Experiments would later observe about a different program, because their deaths would be attributed to their underlying conditions and their objections were unlikely to be effective.

The selection logic was not accidental. It was structural. The people most likely to be defined as raw material were the people least able to resist being used as raw material. That structural logic runs through every program in this book. It begins here.

II. THE LAW

In 1927, the movement reached its American legal apex.

Carrie Buck was eighteen years old. She had been committed to the Virginia State Colony for Epileptics and Feebleminded — a facility whose name reflects its era's institutional vocabulary — after becoming pregnant as the result of rape by a nephew of her foster family. The pregnancy was the stated evidence of her "feeblemindedness." A Eugenics Record Office field worker visited her mother, Emma Buck, at the same institution, and determined that Emma was also feebleminded. The field worker reported that Carrie's infant daughter, Vivian, showed signs of mental defect. Vivian was seven months old.

On the basis of this family record, the state of Virginia sought to sterilize Carrie Buck under its 1924 Eugenical Sterilization Act — a law ERO superintendent Harry Laughlin had helped draft as a model for state legislatures. The case reached the Supreme Court of the United States.

Justice Oliver Wendell Holmes wrote the majority opinion in *Buck v. Bell*, 274 U.S. 200 (1927). The sentence Holmes wrote to justify the decision has never been formally repudiated in American law: "Three generations of imbeciles are enough."

Carrie Buck was sterilized. She lived until 1983. People who knew her in later life described her as an avid reader. Her daughter Vivian, the one whose "mental defect" had been assessed at seven months, made the honor roll at her Charlottesville school before dying of an intestinal disease at age eight.

Buck v. Bell has never been overturned. It remains the law of the United States.

Following the decision, the rate of compulsory sterilizations in American institutions increased sharply. Between 1907 and 1963, over 64,000 individuals were forcibly sterilized under eugenic legislation in the United States across more than thirty states. The state of Virginia did not repeal its sterilization law until 1974. The state of North Carolina issued a formal apology to surviving victims in 2012 and established a compensation program — the only state to do so.

The 64,000 figure is the documented minimum. It counts only the procedures recorded in institutional files that survived. The actual number is unknown.

III. THE GERMAN CONNECTION

The connection between the American eugenics movement and the program that culminated in the Holocaust is documented not in the postwar testimony of survivors but in the correspondence of the American eugenicists themselves, written while the German program was operational.

ERO superintendent Harry Laughlin's model sterilization law — drafted specifically to survive constitutional challenge and tested in the American courts — was implemented in substance in the 1935 Nuremberg racial hygiene legislation. When the University of Heidelberg informed Laughlin of this and offered him an honorary doctorate in recognition of his contribution to "racial hygiene science," he accepted. The correspondence is in the historical record.

California eugenics leader C.M. Goethe wrote to a colleague upon returning from Germany in 1934, where compulsory sterilizations were proceeding at a rate of more than 5,000 per month: "You will be interested to know that your work has played a powerful part in shaping the opinions of the group of intellectuals who are behind Hitler in this epoch-making program. I want you, my dear friend, to carry this thought with you for the rest of your life, that you have really jolted into action a great government of 60 million people."

The Rockefeller Foundation helped establish and fund the Kaiser Wilhelm Institute for Anthropology, Human Heredity, and Eugenics in Berlin — the institution where Josef Mengele conducted research under Otmar von Verschuer before going to Auschwitz. The Foundation's own archives, available through the Rockefeller Archive Center in Sleepy Hollow, New York, document this funding relationship.

When the Nazi doctors were tried at Nuremberg after the war, their defense cited *Buck v. Bell*. They were convicted anyway. But the American legal precedent they cited had not been overturned. The American institutions that had funded the ideology underlying their crimes had not been dissolved.

IV. THE RENAMING

The eugenics movement did not end with the Nazi defeat. It renamed itself.

In 1972, the American Eugenics Society renamed itself the Society for the Study of Social Biology. Its journal, *Eugenics Quarterly*, was renamed *Social Biology*. The rebranding was not accompanied by repudiation of the movement's intellectual premises — it was accompanied by a retreat from the word that had become, after Nuremberg, a liability.

The Carnegie Institution closed the Eugenics Record Office in 1939 as the Nazi connection became publicly damaging. The funding stopped. The ideology did not stop with it.

Historian Edwin Black, whose *War Against the Weak* (Basic Books, 2003) traced the American eugenics movement to its primary sources in exhaustive documented detail, found that scientists who had provided the intellectual architecture for the movement — including Otmar von Verschuer, Mengele's supervisor at the Kaiser Wilhelm Institute, who escaped prosecution after the war — re-established contact with American colleagues. The field rebranded itself as human genetics and population studies. The institutional assumption — that some human beings' biological integrity and reproductive capacity are subject to management by those with the power to manage them — continued to organize research programs, funding structures, and policy recommendations.

The Carnegie Institution closed the ERO. It did not close the assumption the ERO had institutionalized. That assumption traveled forward into the programs this book documents in every subsequent chapter, not because anyone carried it consciously from one program to the next, but because it was already embedded in the institutional culture of American medicine, American research, and American law.

An idea does not need to be remembered to operate. It needs only to have shaped the institutions that outlast it.

V. WHAT THE FOUNDATION BUILT

The practical consequence of the eugenics movement's institutional decades is not only the 64,000 sterilizations. It is the assumption those sterilizations normalized.

Before the eugenics movement, the idea that American institutions had the authority to make irreversible biological decisions about non-consenting citizens — to alter their bodies permanently in the service of a state interest — required justification. After *Buck v. Bell*, it was the law of the land. The Supreme Court had spoken. The Congress had not acted. The president had not objected. The medical profession, whose institutions had been substantially built with the same Rockefeller and Carnegie money that built the Eugenics Record Office, had provided the scientific framework.

The assumption that certain populations — the institutionalized, the imprisoned, the poor, the Black, the Native — were available for biological management without meaningful consent did not need to be re-established for each subsequent program. It was the operating premise. The programs documented in the following chapters — MKUltra, Tuskegee, the radiation experiments, the childhood vaccine schedule's liability shield, the Covid-era hospital protocols — did not import this assumption from outside. They inherited it.

That is what a foundation is for.

PRIMARY SOURCES FOR THIS CHAPTER

- Francis Galton, *Hereditary Genius* (Macmillan, 1869). The founding document of the eugenics movement, available in digitized form through multiple academic repositories including HathiTrust. Galton's argument for the heritability of intelligence and the social management of reproduction is presented in his own words.

- Embryo Project Encyclopedia, "Eugenics Record Office" — embryo.asu.edu. A peer-reviewed reference resource documenting the ERO's founding, funding, operations, and closure, with primary source citations throughout.

- Edwin Black, *War Against the Weak: Eugenics and America's Campaign to Create a Master Race* (Basic Books, 2003; expanded edition Dialog Press, 2012). The most comprehensive documented history of the American eugenics movement, based on primary source research in institutional archives including Carnegie, Rockefeller, and the transferred ERO records now held at the American Philosophical Society in Philadelphia.

- *Buck v. Bell*, 274 U.S. 200 (1927). Full text available at supreme.justia.com and through the Supreme Court's own historical records. Holmes's majority opinion is three pages. The reader is encouraged to read it directly.

- Harry Laughlin, "The Legal Status of Eugenical Sterilization," supplement to the *Annual Report of the Municipal Court of Chicago*, 1929. Laughlin's own documentation of his model sterilization law and its legal standing, cited in the records of the German eugenics program as influential.

- Rockefeller Archive Center, General Education Board and Rockefeller Foundation records, Sleepy Hollow, New York. The primary archive for documentation of Rockefeller funding relationships with both American eugenics institutions and the Kaiser Wilhelm Institute. Open to researchers by appointment.

- Paul A. Lombardo, *Three Generations, No Imbeciles: Eugenics, the Supreme Court, and Buck v. Bell* (Johns Hopkins University Press, 2008). The definitive legal history of the Buck case, documenting the manufactured nature of the evidence and the subsequent lives of Carrie Buck and her daughter Vivian.

The primary sources for this chapter are in institutional archives, published books, and the Supreme Court's own record. None of them require the reader to trust an advocacy organization. They require only the willingness to read what the principals wrote and what the courts decided.

Chapter 2: The Medical Capture

The Flexner Report, the Pharmaceutical Monopoly, and the Elimination of the Competition

"Is there no balm in Gilead? Is there no physician there? Why then has the health of the daughter of my people not been restored?"

— Jeremiah 8:22

The prophet is asking about healing that should exist and does not. He is not asking about ignorance — the balm of Gilead was real, the physicians were real, the tradition of healing was real. He is asking about a failure of a different kind: the systematic unavailability of what should have been available, to the people who most needed it.

The question is twenty-six centuries old. It describes the American medical system of the twenty-first century with a precision that should be uncomfortable.

In 1910 — the same year the Eugenics Record Office was established at Cold Spring Harbor — a document was published that would restructure American medicine more thoroughly than any legislation in the country's history. It was not a law. It was a report. Its author was Abraham Flexner, an educator with no medical degree, no clinical experience, and no independent standing in the profession he was about to transform.

What he had was the backing of Andrew Carnegie.

I. THE REPORT AND ITS SPONSOR

The document was called *Medical Education in the United States and Canada: A Report to the Carnegie Foundation for the Advancement of Teaching*. Flexner had visited 155 American and Canadian medical schools over the preceding eighteen months, evaluating each against a single standard: the Johns Hopkins School of Medicine, with its emphasis on laboratory science, germ theory, and pharmaceutical pharmacology. Schools that matched the Hopkins model were rated adequate. Schools that did not — those teaching botanical medicine, homeopathy, naturopathy, electrotherapy, and the other clinical traditions that had occupied legitimate positions in American healing — were characterized as substandard, dangerous, and unworthy of continued operation.

The Flexner Report itself is a public document. It is available through the Carnegie Foundation archives and through HathiTrust's digital repository. The reader who goes to the primary source will find a document that reads as a scientific assessment but functions as a blueprint for market consolidation. The schools Flexner praised were schools organized around the pharmaceutical model — the model in which treatment means the administration of patented synthetic compounds produced by the chemical industry. The schools he condemned were schools teaching traditions of healing that did not require those products.

The funding mechanism that converted the report's recommendations into institutional reality was the Rockefeller-funded General Education Board — the same philanthropic vehicle that had helped fund the eugenics movement. The GEB directed its medical education grants to schools that aligned with the pharmaceutical model. It withheld grants from those that did not. No law required the competing schools to close. The money was sufficient.

By 1935, the number of American medical schools had declined from 155 to 66. The schools that survived were those teaching pharmaceutical medicine. The schools that closed were those teaching the competing traditions — including, disproportionately, the schools that had served Black communities and women, populations the surviving schools largely excluded. The consolidation was not only medical. It was social.

II. WHO FUNDED WHOM

The connection between the men who funded the Flexner Report and the men who stood to profit from its implementation is direct and documented.

John D. Rockefeller's Standard Oil fortune had been partially reinvested in the pharmaceutical and chemical industries. The General Education Board, which Rockefeller had endowed with more than $180 million by 1920, directed medical education grants in ways that systematically advantaged schools teaching medicine organized around pharmaceutical products — the products of the industries in which Rockefeller capital was invested. E. Richard Brown's *Rockefeller Medicine Men* (University of California Press, 1979) traces these funding relationships through primary source documentation from the Rockefeller Archive Center, demonstrating that the GEB's grant decisions were not neutral assessments of educational quality but strategic investments in a particular model of medicine — the model that required the products Rockefeller's other investments produced.

This is not conspiracy. It is the ordinary operation of capital seeking to consolidate the institutional conditions for its own reproduction. The pharmaceutical monopoly was not the result of a secret plan. It was the result of the systematic application of money to the question of which traditions of healing would survive and which would not.

Paul Starr's *The Social Transformation of American Medicine* (Basic Books, 1982), which won the Pulitzer Prize in 1984, documents the professionalization process and the consolidation of medical authority in the language of mainstream American sociology. Starr's account is not hostile to the institutions he describes. It is careful, documented, and credentialed. And it shows, without intending this as an indictment, how thoroughly the structure of American medicine was reshaped in the decades following the Flexner Report — not by scientific discovery but by the decisions of private philanthropic institutions acting in alignment with their economic interests.

III. WHAT WAS ELIMINATED

The traditions the Flexner Report characterized as substandard were not simply inferior versions of pharmaceutical medicine. They were different approaches to the same question — what does a sick human being need to recover? — organized around different assumptions about the nature of the body and the nature of healing.

Botanical medicine worked with the body's own regulatory systems, using plant compounds that human beings had been using for healing across millennia, refined by clinical experience across cultures and generations. Homeopathy worked on the principle of like curing like and had its own clinical tradition. Naturopathy emphasized the body's inherent healing capacity and the role of nutrition, rest, and environmental conditions. Osteopathy worked with the musculoskeletal system's relationship to organ function. Midwifery served the vast majority of American births.

These traditions shared something the pharmaceutical model did not: they did not require the ongoing purchase of patented synthetic products to function. A physician practicing botanical medicine could use plants that grew locally. A midwife carried knowledge, not inventory. The healing tradition that does not require a supply chain is a tradition that does not produce a revenue stream for the investor who has capitalized the supply chain.

That is not a sufficient reason to eliminate a tradition of healing. It was, in practice, what happened.

After the Flexner restructuring, physicians trained in the surviving schools were not taught botanical medicine, homeopathy, or nutrition as primary clinical tools. They were taught pharmacology — the science of drug action — as the core of their clinical practice. Subsequent generations of physicians were not taught the eliminated traditions at all. They learned that those traditions were unscientific, not because the clinical evidence had been carefully evaluated and found wanting, but because the institutional structure of medical education had made them invisible. You cannot learn a tradition that is no longer taught.

The word that names what was done — and that gives this book its title — is not metaphor. The animal in the pen is not taught to find its own food. Its food is provided. Its health is managed. Its productivity is harvested. The patient produced by the Flexner restructuring inhabits a medical system whose economic health depends on the patient's continued dependence on its products. That dependence is most reliably produced not by curing disease but by managing its symptoms indefinitely — by turning acute conditions into chronic ones, and by ensuring that the chronic conditions are addressed by interventions that can be owned, patented, and sold at whatever price the absence of competition permits.

IV. THE STRUCTURAL CONSEQUENCE

The practical consequence of the Flexner restructuring, fully realized across the following century, is the American chronic disease epidemic.

As of the most recent CDC data, six in ten American adults have at least one chronic disease. Four in ten have two or more. Obesity affects more than 40 percent of American adults. Type 2 diabetes affects more than 37 million Americans. Heart disease remains the leading cause of death. Autoimmune conditions affect an estimated 23 million Americans, a figure the NIH itself has characterized as likely an underestimate. The United States spends more on healthcare per capita than any other high-income nation and produces worse population health outcomes than most of them on nearly every measurable dimension.

This is not a failure of the pharmaceutical model. It is the pharmaceutical model operating as its institutional incentives predict it will operate. A system whose revenue depends on the ongoing management of chronic conditions does not have an economic incentive to prevent or cure those conditions. The system functions exactly as the incentive structure that the Flexner restructuring established would predict.

The reader who objects that individual physicians within the system are genuinely motivated to help their patients — this is true and is not in dispute. The individual physician's motivation and the system's institutional incentive are different things. Most physicians who followed the ventilator protocols in 2020, as Chapter 12 will document, were following institutional guidelines while genuinely trying to help their patients. The institutional incentive and the individual intention can point in different directions. When they do, in a captured system, the institutional incentive wins.

The Flexner restructuring did not create the pharmaceutical monopoly alone. It created the institutional monopoly that made the pharmaceutical capture of medicine structurally inevitable. The consolidated medical school system, funded by Rockefeller and Carnegie money and oriented around pharmaceutical pharmacology, produced generations of physicians who had no framework for healing outside the product model. Those physicians populated the regulatory agencies, the professional societies, the hospital administrations, and the insurance structures that now govern American medicine. They were not corrupted. They were trained.

V. THE SPECIFIC YEAR

One detail is worth holding: 1910.

The Eugenics Record Office was established at Cold Spring Harbor in 1910. The Flexner Report was published in 1910. The same philanthropic network — Carnegie, Rockefeller — funded both. The same year that institutionalized the idea that some human beings are raw material to be managed also institutionalized the medical system through which they would be managed.

This is not an argument for conspiracy between the eugenics movement and the Flexner restructuring. It is an observation about whose money was building the institutional architecture of American biological management in the first decade of the twentieth century, and what that architecture, taken as a whole, was designed to produce.

The eugenics movement established the ideological premise: some bodies exist to be managed. The Flexner restructuring established the institutional mechanism: a consolidated medical authority whose economic health depends on managing them. The chapters that follow document how that premise and that mechanism operated in practice, on specific populations, in specific programs, across the following century.

Jeremiah's question — why has the health of my people not been restored? — is not rhetorical in the prophet's text. He knows the answer. The balm is real. The physicians exist. The failure is not ignorance. It is something else: the calculated unavailability of what would heal, in the service of interests that benefit from the continuation of the wound.

PRIMARY SOURCES FOR THIS CHAPTER

- Abraham Flexner, *Medical Education in the United States and Canada*, Carnegie Foundation for the Advancement of Teaching, Bulletin Number Four, 1910. Full text available digitally through the Carnegie Foundation archives and through HathiTrust (catalog.hathitrust.org). The reader who reads the primary document will find the evaluative criteria and the specific recommendations in Flexner's own language.

- Rockefeller Archive Center, General Education Board records, Sleepy Hollow, New York. The primary archive for documentation of GEB grant decisions and the funding relationships between Rockefeller philanthropy and pharmaceutical-aligned medical schools. Open to researchers. Finding aids available online at rockarch.org.

- Paul Starr, *The Social Transformation of American Medicine* (Basic Books, 1982). Pulitzer Prize-winning sociological history of American medicine's professionalization, documenting the consolidation of institutional authority and the decline of competing traditions with extensive primary source citation.

- E. Richard Brown, *Rockefeller Medicine Men: Medicine and Capitalism in America* (University of California Press, 1979). The most direct documented account of the relationship between Rockefeller capital and the restructuring of American medicine, drawing on primary sources from the Rockefeller Archive Center.

- Bonner, Thomas Neville, *Iconoclast: Abraham Flexner and a Life in Learning* (Johns Hopkins University Press, 2002). The standard biographical treatment of Flexner, useful for establishing his background, his Carnegie relationship, and the context of the report's production.

- Centers for Disease Control and Prevention, "Chronic Diseases in America" — cdc.gov/chronicdisease. The CDC's own summary of chronic disease prevalence in the United States, providing current population-level data on the outcomes of the system the Flexner restructuring produced.

The Flexner Report is available online. The Rockefeller Archive is open to researchers. The chronic disease statistics are on the CDC's website. Every claim in this chapter is verifiable from documents that require no special access to obtain. The reader is encouraged to start with the Report itself — available in its entirety, free, at HathiTrust — and read what Flexner actually wrote about the schools he was condemning.

Chapter 3: The Transfer

Operation Paperclip and the Importation of the Experimental Ideology

"Truly, I say to you, as you did it to one of the least of these my brothers, you did it to me."

— Matthew 25:40

On May 8, 1945, Germany surrendered. Six weeks later, the United States government began a program to recruit the scientists who had built the Nazi war machine and bring them to America.

What the program transferred was not only technical knowledge. It was an ideology: that human beings — specifically, certain categories of human beings — are available as experimental subjects when the institutional interest is sufficiently important. That availability does not require consent. It does not require that the subject understand what is being done to them. It requires only that the subject be accessible and that the institution have the power to use them.

Chapter 1 documented the American roots of this ideology in the eugenics movement. Chapter 2 documented the institutional mechanism — the consolidated medical authority — through which it would operate. This chapter documents the importation, in 1945, of its most systematic institutional expression: the Nazi experimental program's ideology, carried across the Atlantic by more than 1,600 scientists whose records had been altered to conceal what they had done and who they had been.

The verse that opens this chapter is not placed for rhetorical effect. The people who would be used in the programs the transferred ideology produced — the subjects of MKUltra, the men of Tuskegee, the patients at Cincinnati General — are the people

Jesus named as his own presence in the world. What was done to them was done to him. The chapter that follows this one documents what was done.

I. THE PROGRAM AND ITS RECORD

The program that became known as Operation Paperclip was formally initiated by the U.S. Joint Chiefs of Staff on July 20, 1945. Its stated purpose was to exploit German scientific and technical expertise for the ongoing war against Japan and to strengthen American postwar military and industrial research. Its operational mechanism was the Joint Intelligence Objectives Agency — the JIOA — whose function was to identify, recruit, and resettle German scientists in the United States.

The JIOA's personnel dossiers on more than 1,500 German and Austrian scientists are held today in the National Archives in Washington, D.C., in Record Group 330. They are available to researchers. Annie Jacobsen's *Operation Paperclip* (Little, Brown, 2014) drew extensively on these records, as did Linda Hunt's earlier *Secret Agenda* (St. Martin's Press, 1991). The Advisory Committee on Human Radiation Experiments reviewed the JIOA records specifically in connection with Paperclip scientists who went on to conduct radiation experiments on non-consenting American citizens, and its findings are available through the Department of Energy's OpenNet system.

President Harry Truman had explicitly prohibited the recruitment of active Nazi supporters. The JIOA's solution, documented in its own records, was to alter the dossiers — removing, in the language of program critics, evidence of Nazi Party membership, SS affiliation, and in some cases participation in programs that had used concentration camp prisoners as experimental subjects. The word used in program documentation for this process was "exploitation." The scientists were being exploited for American purposes. Their records were being exploited to make the recruitment possible.

JIOA director Navy Captain Bosquet Wev put the operational logic plainly in an April 27, 1948 memo to the Pentagon's Director of Intelligence. He wrote that security investigations had found that the majority of recruited German scientists had been members of the Nazi Party or its affiliates, but characterized this as the product of ordinary social pressure rather than ideological commitment. He was critical of what he considered over-scrupulous investigations by the Department of Justice. His memo is in the National Archives. You can read it.

II. THE NAMED CASES

More than 1,600 scientists ultimately came to the United States under Paperclip and related programs. The individual cases most relevant to the lineage this book documents are not primarily the rocket engineers — von Braun and his colleagues at Peenemünde — though they are the most famous. They are the biomedical researchers.

Wernher von Braun is included because his case establishes the pattern. Von Braun was an SS officer. His V-2 program used approximately 60,000 slave laborers from the Mittelbau-Dora concentration camp — a satellite of Buchenwald — to manufacture rockets in underground tunnels. The death rate among workers at Mittelbau-Dora exceeded the number of people killed by the V-2s themselves. Von Braun knew where his labor came from. He visited the facility. After Paperclip, he became the director of NASA's Marshall Space Flight Center and the public face of the American space program. His face appeared on the cover of Time magazine. He received the National Medal of Science.

Hubertus Strughold was the director of the Luftwaffe's Aeromedical Research Institute during the war. His institute's research included experiments on human subjects at high altitude and in freezing water — experiments conducted on concentration camp prisoners at Dachau. After Paperclip, Strughold built a distinguished American career at the School of Aerospace Medicine in San Antonio, Texas, and became known as the "father of space medicine." In 1963, the Space Medicine Branch of the Aerospace Medical Association established the Hubertus Strughold Award, given annually to outstanding contributors in the field. The award was rescinded in 2013 after historians documented his wartime record more fully.

Kurt Blome was the Nazi Deputy Surgeon General and a senior official in the program that developed biological weapons. He was tried at the Nuremberg Doctors' Trial and acquitted. Shortly after his acquittal, he was recruited by the U.S. Army Chemical Corps for consultation on biological weapons research. The Advisory Committee on Human Radiation Experiments documented his recruitment and his subsequent work in the American research apparatus.

These individual cases are important but not primary. What matters for the lineage this book documents is what they collectively represent.

III. THE IDEOLOGY THAT TRAVELED

The Nazi experimental program had developed the non-consensual human experiment to its most systematic institutional expression. This is what distinguished it from the American eugenics programs documented in Chapter 1, which operated primarily through coercion and exclusion. The Nazi program added the assembly-line experimental methodology: the deliberate, meticulous, documented use of identified populations — prisoners, Jews,

Roma, the disabled, Soviet POWs — as experimental subjects in programs designed to answer questions of military and industrial utility, without any pretense of therapeutic benefit to the subjects.

The Nuremberg Code, adopted in 1947 specifically in response to the evidence presented at the Doctors' Trial, stated its first principle with the clarity that atrocity demands: "The voluntary consent of the human subject is absolutely essential." The Code continued: consent means the subject "should have sufficient knowledge and comprehension of the elements of the subject matter involved as to enable him to make an understanding and enlightened decision." No deception. No coercion. No substitution of institutional judgment for individual choice.

Paperclip began in 1945. The Nuremberg Code was adopted in 1947. Operation Paperclip predated the Code by two years — but the Doctors' Trial, at which the evidence that produced the Code was presented, ran from December 1946 through August 1947. American researchers and intelligence officials who had recruited Paperclip scientists were aware of the Doctors' Trial and its findings. The Code was adopted in explicit response to the experimental methodology the American government had simultaneously imported.

Within years of the Code's adoption, American researchers were violating it on American soil.

The Advisory Committee on Human Radiation Experiments, reviewing the government's own records in 1994 and 1995, found that several Paperclip scientists went on to conduct or advise on radiation experiments involving non-consenting American subjects. The committee's *Final Report* is careful to distinguish between the specific Paperclip scientists whose American research records raised questions and the broader population of 1,600 scientists, most of whom had no documented connection to human experimentation. But the committee's broader finding is the relevant one for this book: that a culture had developed in the American research apparatus, in the years immediately following Paperclip, in which the use of non-consenting subjects was accepted practice — and that the Paperclip transfer had introduced into that apparatus scientists who had operated within an institutional culture where this practice was not only accepted but systematized.

An ideology does not travel in a briefcase. It travels in the assumptions of the people who hold it — in what they consider normal, in what institutional practices they recognize as legitimate, in what populations they recognize as available for use. The people who came through Paperclip brought with them, among other things, a set of assumptions about the relationship between the researcher and the subject. Those assumptions did not arrive labeled as such. They arrived as professional practice, as methodological precedent, as the normal operating procedures of people who had worked in a specific institutional culture.

That is how ideologies travel. That is how this one did.

IV. THE NUREMBERG CODE AND WHAT FOLLOWED

It is worth being precise about the timeline.

1945: Operation Paperclip begins. More than 1,600 German scientists are recruited to the United States, their records altered to facilitate immigration.

1946–1947: The Nuremberg Doctors' Trial documents the Nazi experimental program. Twenty of the twenty-three defendants are found guilty. Seven are executed. The Nuremberg Code is adopted as the international standard for ethical human experimentation.

1947: The Nuremberg Code's first principle states that voluntary informed consent is "absolutely essential."

1950: The first experiments of what will become the MKUltra program are conducted by the CIA's predecessor organization, the Office of Strategic Services, on non-consenting subjects.

1953: MKUltra is formally established by CIA Director Allen Dulles.

1956: The FBI's COINTELPRO program begins systematic operations targeting domestic political organizations.

1932–1972: The Tuskegee syphilis study runs — begun before the Nuremberg Code, continuing for twenty-five years after it.

The timeline is not complicated. The people who built the Nuremberg Code and the people who violated it were operating in the same institutional environment, in the same country, at the same time. The Code did not create an era of ethical human experimentation in American research. It created an era of ethical rhetoric about human experimentation, behind which the programs documented in the following chapters operated.

The subjects of those programs are who they are. The verse above names them. The programs did what they did. The verse names what that means.

PRIMARY SOURCES FOR THIS CHAPTER

- National Archives, Record Group 330, JIOA personnel dossiers, Washington D.C. The primary operational record of Operation Paperclip, including the dossiers on individual scientists, the correspondence between JIOA and other government agencies, and the documentation of the record-alteration process. Available to researchers; finding aids at archives.gov.

- JIOA Director Bosquet Wev, memorandum to the Director of Intelligence, Department of the Army, April 27, 1948. Reproduced and cited in multiple published accounts of Paperclip, and available through the National Archives records.

- Advisory Committee on Human Radiation Experiments, *Final Report* (U.S. Government Printing Office, 1995), particularly Tab F-3 on Operation Paperclip scientists in the American research apparatus. Available through the Department of Energy's OpenNet system at opennet.energy.gov, reference 16385196.

- Annie Jacobsen, *Operation Paperclip: The Secret Intelligence Program that Brought Nazi Scientists to America* (Little, Brown, 2014). Draws directly on the JIOA records in the National Archives, with documentation for every named case. The most comprehensive and sourced account of the program currently available.

- Linda Hunt, *Secret Agenda: The United States Government, Nazi Scientists, and Project Paperclip, 1945 to 1990* (St. Martin's Press, 1991). Earlier documented account of the program, drawing on declassified government records.

- Nuremberg Code (1947), reproduced in full in *Trials of War Criminals Before the Nuremberg Military Tribunals Under Control Council Law No. 10*, Volume II (U.S. Government Printing Office, 1949–1953). The Code's ten principles are available through numerous primary source archives and through the U.S. Holocaust Memorial Museum at ushmm.org.

- Nazi War Crimes and Japanese Imperial Government Records Interagency Working Group, declassified records on Operation Paperclip, available through archives.gov/iwg. Congressional mandate produced additional declassification of Paperclip-related records in the late 1990s and early 2000s.

Every scientist named in this chapter is named in primary source documents available in the National Archives, in the ACHRE Final Report, or in both. Nothing in this chapter is based on secondary assertion. The reader who wants to verify the cases of von Braun, Strughold, or Blome is directed to the National Archives records and to the ACHRE Final Report, which cites the primary documents throughout.

Chapter 4: MKUltra

The CIA, Non-Consent, and the Assault on the Human Mind

"For God gave us a spirit not of fear but of power and love and self-control."

— 2 Timothy 1:7

The verse names three faculties. Power: the capacity to act from one's own will. Love: the capacity to extend the self toward another. Self-control: the capacity to govern one's own responses, to choose rather than to react, to be the author of one's own behavior rather than its subject.

These are the faculties the MKUltra program was specifically designed to destroy.

Not incidentally. Not as a side effect. As the program's stated operational objective. The CIA's own documents — approximately 20,000 of them, surviving only because they were misfiled in a financial records building and escaped the 1973 destruction order — describe a systematic effort to break the human mind's capacity for autonomous self-direction, to erase individual identity, and to rewrite human behavior through a combination of pharmacological assault, psychological torture, sensory deprivation, and hypnosis.

The Nuremberg Code had been adopted six years before the program began. The people who designed MKUltra knew the Code. They knew what it said. They proceeded in calculated rejection of it.

This chapter documents what they did, in their own words, from the surviving record.

I. THE PROGRAM: SCOPE AND ORIGINS

On August 3, 1977, Admiral Stansfield Turner, Director of the Central Intelligence Agency, testified before the joint session of the Senate Select Committee on Intelligence and the Subcommittee on Health and Scientific Research. The hearing was titled "Project MKULTRA: The CIA's Program of Research in Behavioral Modification." Turner acknowledged, under oath and before the Senate, that the CIA had conducted the program across 80 institutions — 44 colleges and universities, 15 research foundations, 12 hospitals and clinics, and 3 prisons — through 149 separately funded research projects. The hearing transcript, including Turner's testimony and the documents entered into the congressional record, is available through the Senate archives.

The program had been formally established in 1953 by CIA Director Allen Dulles under the code name MKULTRA. It was the continuation and expansion of predecessor programs — ARTICHOKE and BLUEBIRD — that had begun as early as 1950 in the CIA's predecessor organization, the Office of Strategic Services. The stated rationale was the Cold War: the belief that the Soviet Union and China had developed techniques of behavioral control through their handling of American prisoners of war in Korea, and that the United States needed both countermeasures and matching capabilities.

The Cold War rationale is documented. So is the fact that the program's experiments produced no validated scientific findings that advanced either goal. Historian John Marks, whose *The Search for the Manchurian Candidate* (Times Books, 1979) remains the foundational documented account of MKUltra, reviewed the surviving documents after obtaining them through a Freedom of Information Act request and found that the program's research was operationally motivated rather than scientifically driven — designed not to produce knowledge but to develop tools.

The tool was a controllable human being. The program never produced one.

What it did produce, across more than two decades of operation, is documented in the surviving files.

II. THE METHODS

The program's methods fall into several documented categories.

Pharmacological assault. LSD was the primary tool. The drug was administered to subjects without their knowledge or consent — dissolved in drinks, administered in injections described as vitamins or medical treatments, given in what subjects were told were routine experimental procedures of other kinds. The operational objective was not recreation or therapy. It was the disruption of the subject's psychological defenses and the creation of a state of maximum suggestibility. CIA documents describe the goal as accessing "the innermost recesses of the human mind" — the territory below conscious control, where, the program's designers believed, behavior could be reprogrammed.

The doses administered were not recreational doses. They were doses calculated to produce extreme psychological disorientation. Subjects who did not know they had been given a psychedelic drug — who had no framework for interpreting what was happening to their perception and cognition — experienced what they could only understand as mental breakdown. Some did not recover.

Sensory deprivation. Extended periods of isolation, darkness, silence, or continuous white noise were used to break down the subject's sense of self and reality. The program's documents describe these techniques in clinical language. The experience they produced in human beings was terror and psychological dissolution.

Hypnosis. The program extensively investigated hypnosis as a method of behavioral control — the creation of post-hypnotic suggestions, the implantation of false memories, the establishment of behavioral triggers that could be activated remotely. The operational ambition was the controllable agent: a person who could be directed to perform a specific action, including violence, without conscious awareness of having been directed.

Psychological torture. The program drew explicitly on techniques documented in the Nazi experimental literature — including research conducted at Dachau and other concentration camps on the effects of extreme stress, cold, and pain on human psychology. The Paperclip scientists who had entered the American research apparatus after 1945, and the institutional culture they had helped establish, were part of the knowledge base the program's designers drew on.

III. THE SUBJECTS

The populations selected for MKUltra experiments were selected on the same logic documented in Chapter 1: they were people whose objections were unlikely to be effective and whose psychological distress was unlikely to be attributed to anything other than their underlying conditions.

Prisoners were used in experiments at federal penitentiaries — people whose institutional confinement gave them no meaningful ability to refuse. Psychiatric patients were used in hospitals that served as CIA operational fronts — people whose reports of what was being done to them would be dismissed as symptoms of their conditions. Drug addicts were used in a CIA safe house in San Francisco, where, in an operation called MIDNIGHT CLIMAX, subjects were dosed with LSD by CIA-employed prostitutes while agents observed through one-way mirrors. Soldiers were used in military experiments — people under institutional command structures that made refusal insubordination. Foreign nationals were used in experiments conducted overseas, beyond the reach of whatever domestic legal constraints nominally applied.

The people who could not say no were the people used. This is not inference. It is in the program's own operational rationale, documented in the surviving files and in the testimony of CIA officials before the Senate.

The most extensively documented subprogram was conducted at McGill University's Allen Memorial Institute in Montreal, by Dr. Ewen Cameron. Cameron served simultaneously as president of the American Psychiatric Association, the Canadian Psychiatric Association, and the World Psychiatric Association — the most credentialed institutional positions in psychiatry, on two continents, simultaneously. He received CIA funding through a front organization called the Society for the Investigation of Human Ecology.

His experiments — which he called "psychic driving" — were conducted on psychiatric patients who had come to him for treatment of ordinary conditions: anxiety, mild depression, marital problems. They did not consent to what was done to them. Cameron administered massive doses of electroconvulsive therapy — sometimes 30 to 40 times in a single day, far beyond any therapeutic application — combined with drug-induced sleep for periods of weeks or months, sensory deprivation, and continuous tape-recorded messages played on loops designed to erase and rewrite behavior.

He called the process "depatterning." The goal was to reduce the patient to a pre-verbal, pre-cognitive state — to erase the adult personality entirely — and then use the recorded messages to install a new behavioral pattern. The process did not work as Cameron intended. What it produced was permanent psychological damage. Patients who had come to him for help with moderate conditions left with destroyed memories, lost decades of their lives, regressed to infantile states, and lost the cognitive function they had come with intact. Some never recovered.

Cameron's funding from the CIA front organization was documented by journalist John Marks in the FOIA-released files. His Canadian victims subsequently filed suit against the Canadian government, which had also provided him with funding. The Canadian government settled. His American victims filed suit against the CIA. The case was settled out of court in 1988. The settlements are documented. Cameron died in 1967 and was never prosecuted.

IV. THE DESTRUCTION AND WHAT SURVIVED

In January 1973, CIA Director Richard Helms ordered the destruction of the MKUltra files before a potential congressional investigation could access them. The destruction was carried out. Most of the program's records — an unknown but certainly substantial quantity of documentation — was permanently lost.

What survived was approximately 20,000 documents, misfiled in a CIA financial records building in Rockville, Maryland, that was not included in the destruction order. These documents were discovered in 1977 during a routine audit, sought through a FOIA request by journalist John Marks, and released — with significant redactions — to form the documented basis of the Senate hearing and of Marks's subsequent book.

The decision to destroy the files is itself documented. It is in the congressional record. Richard Helms, when asked about it before the Senate, acknowledged ordering the destruction. He was not prosecuted for it. The deliberate destruction of federal records is a federal crime. In the case of MKUltra, it was the senior official of one of the nation's primary intelligence agencies, and the consequence was no consequence.

The reader who remembers Chapter 13's account of David Morens instructing colleagues on how to make emails "disappear" in 2021 will recognize the operating principle. The specific technology for destroying the record changes across generations. The institutional impulse to destroy it does not.

V. THE CONSEQUENCE AND THE COVER

The 1977 Senate hearing was not the first time Congress had looked at MKUltra. The Church Committee, investigating domestic intelligence abuses in 1975 and 1976, had touched on the program. Senator Frank Church had expressed alarm. The senators who heard Turner's 1977 testimony expressed more alarm.

No legislation creating criminal penalties for those who authorized or conducted the experiments was passed. No researcher who had subjected non-consenting human beings to pharmacological assault and psychological torture was prosecuted. The institutions that had served as CIA operational fronts — the universities, the hospitals, the research foundations — were not dissolved. They received no meaningful institutional sanction. Many are still operating, still receiving federal research funding.

The Frank Olson case illuminates why meaningful accountability was structurally unavailable. Olson was a biological weapons researcher at Fort Detrick, Maryland — a senior government scientist with security clearances and institutional standing. In November 1953, he was dosed with LSD without his knowledge or consent by his CIA handlers during a team meeting at a rural Maryland retreat. Nine days later, he fell from the window of a New York hotel room on the thirteenth floor and died. The death was ruled a suicide.

In 1994, Olson's family had his body exhumed. Forensic

examination found evidence of blunt force trauma to the head inconsistent with a fall. A New York medical examiner concluded the manner of death was "undetermined" rather than suicide. Eric Olson, Frank's son, has spent decades pursuing the case. The U.S. government settled a wrongful death suit with the family in 1976. The settlement is documented. The full circumstances of Frank Olson's death have not been established in any court proceeding.

The case matters not primarily as a crime story but as an illustration of what MKUltra's operational culture produced. A senior government scientist was drugged without his consent at a team meeting by the people he worked with. When he became psychologically destabilized in the days that followed, the people responsible for his destabilization managed his response — contained him, monitored him, decided what would happen to him — rather than getting him help. And then he went out a hotel window.

That is what an institution looks like when the assumption that some people are available for use without consent has been fully operational long enough to become invisible. You do not think of it as wrong. You think of it as operational necessity.

PRIMARY SOURCES FOR THIS CHAPTER

- United States Senate Select Committee on Intelligence and the Subcommittee on Health and Scientific Research, "Project MKULTRA: The CIA's Program of Research in Behavioral Modification," Joint Hearing, August 3, 1977. Full transcript including CIA Director Stansfield Turner's testimony and the documents entered into the record. Available through the Senate historical archives and reproduced at the National Security Archive at George Washington University (nsarchive.gwu.edu).

- National Security Archive, George Washington University, MKUltra documents collection. The surviving FOIA-released documents, with finding aids. Available at nsarchive.gwu.edu/project/mkultra-vault.

- John Marks, *The Search for the Manchurian Candidate: The CIA and Mind Control* (Times Books, 1979; Norton paperback, 1991). The foundational documented account of MKUltra, based on the FOIA-released documents. Marks obtained the documents; his book is organized around them and cites them throughout.

- Church Committee, United States Senate Select Committee to Study Governmental Operations with Respect to Intelligence Activities, *Final Report, Book I: Foreign and Military Intelligence* and *Book II: Intelligence Activities and the Rights of Americans* (U.S. Government Printing Office, 1976). Available through the Senate Historical Office. MKUltra appears in multiple contexts throughout the investigation.

- H.P. Albarelli Jr., *A Terrible Mistake: The Murder of Frank Olson and the CIA's Secret Cold War Experiments* (Trine Day, 2009). The most exhaustive documented investigation of the Olson case, drawing on FOIA-released CIA records, interviews, and the forensic findings from the 1994 exhumation.

- Canadian government documentation of Ewen Cameron's experiments and the subsequent settlement with Canadian victims of the Montreal experiments. Documented in Canadian parliamentary records and in reporting by the CBC and *The Globe and Mail*, drawing on government records released in Canada.

- Nuremberg Code (1947). The Code is reproduced in full in *Trials of War Criminals Before the Nuremberg Military Tribunals*, Volume II, available through the U.S. Holocaust Memorial Museum at ushmm.org. Its ten principles, including the first principle on voluntary consent, are available in multiple primary source archives.

The Senate hearing transcript of August 3, 1977 is the primary document for this chapter. It is in the public record. Admiral Turner's testimony and the documents entered into the record establish, in the CIA's own acknowledged account, the scope, the methods, and the institutional structure of MKUltra. Everything else in this chapter is sourced from documents that flow from that foundational primary record. The reader is directed there first.

Chapter 5: The Domestic Parallel

Tuskegee, the Radiation Experiments, and the Native Assumption

"Open your mouth for the mute, for the rights of all who are destitute. Open your mouth, judge righteously, defend the poor and needy."

— Proverbs 31:8–9

The previous chapter documented MKUltra. This chapter exists because of a specific argument that follows MKUltra in almost every public discussion of it: that programs like that represent aberrations — the behavior of a specific agency, in a specific Cold War context, that does not reflect the broader American research culture. The argument has a specific corollary: that the ideology of non-consensual human experimentation was imported through Operation Paperclip, and that without the German transfer documented in Chapter 3, American research would not have gone there.

This chapter refutes both arguments with primary source documentation.

The two programs documented below required no German input. They were conceived, funded, staffed, and operated by American institutions, using American funding, on American soil, under American law. The people who conducted them were not Nazi scientists imported under altered dossiers. They were American physicians, American public health officials, American university researchers — people working within the normal institutional structures of American medicine and American science.

The ideology that made what they did possible was not imported. It was native.

I. TUSKEGEE: FORTY YEARS

In 1932, the United States Public Health Service launched a study of untreated syphilis in Black men in Macon County, Alabama. The study enrolled 399 men with syphilis and 201 uninfected controls. The men were told they were receiving treatment for "bad blood" — a local term covering a range of conditions. They were not told they had syphilis. They were not given treatment for syphilis.

When penicillin became the accepted cure for syphilis in 1947 — the year the Nuremberg Code was adopted — the study continued. The decision was made explicitly not to treat the men with penicillin. The reasoning, documented in the study's own internal records: treating them would end the study. The study's value to the researchers was in observing untreated syphilis in its natural progression over time. Treatment would interrupt the observation. The observation was considered more important than the men.

The study ran for forty years.

It was ended in 1972 not by internal institutional review, not by a physician who objected and was heard, not by a regulatory agency that discovered the protocol and intervened. It was ended when a Public Health Service employee named Peter Buxtun leaked information about it to journalist Jean Heller, whose story appeared simultaneously in newspapers across the country on July 25, 1972. Congress held hearings. A panel determined the study had been "ethically unjustifiable." The study was terminated.

The panel's most important finding, rarely quoted in full, was that the researchers were not ignorant of the ethical frameworks that prohibited what they were doing. The Nuremberg Code had been adopted twenty-five years before the panel met. The Declaration of Helsinki — the World Medical Association's codification of research ethics — had been adopted in 1964. The researchers had access to these frameworks. They had simply applied them differently to the population they were studying than they would have applied them to any other population.

The documented human cost, by the time the study ended: 28 men had died of syphilis directly. 100 had died of related complications. 40 wives had been infected. 19 children had been born with congenital syphilis. All of this was preventable from 1947 onward — the moment penicillin became available — and was not prevented because prevention would have ended the study.

The study's findings had been published throughout its forty-year operation in mainstream peer-reviewed medical journals, including the *Journal of Chronic Diseases* and *Venereal Disease Information*. These publications are in the National Library of Medicine's archive. They were not hidden. Other physicians read them. They appeared at conferences. The study was not a secret program. It was an open publication record of a forty-year experiment on men who did not know they were experimental subjects.

No researcher who conducted the study was prosecuted. No institution that funded or hosted it was dissolved. President Clinton issued a formal apology to the surviving participants in 1997. The apology is in the public record.

James H. Jones's *Bad Blood: The Tuskegee Syphilis Experiment* (Free Press, 1981; expanded 1993) is the definitive documented history of the study, drawing on the Public Health Service's own records and the congressional investigation files. The reader who wants to understand what the researchers actually wrote about what they were doing — in their own published papers, in their own internal memos — will find it in Jones's account, sourced throughout.

II. THE RADIATION EXPERIMENTS: THOUSANDS

In 1994, President Clinton established the Advisory Committee on Human Radiation Experiments, directed by executive order to investigate allegations that the U.S. government had conducted radiation experiments on non-consenting subjects during and after World War II. The committee's *Final Report*, published in 1995 by the U.S. Government Printing Office, is available through the Department of Energy's OpenNet system. It is 925 pages long. It is exhaustively sourced. Everything that follows is drawn from it.

The committee identified thousands of experiments conducted on hundreds of thousands of subjects at institutions that included the University of Chicago, the University of California, Vanderbilt University, Ohio State University, and Cincinnati General Hospital. The experiments were funded by the Atomic Energy Commission, the Department of Defense, and the National Institutes of Health. The researchers who conducted them were not peripheral figures in American science. They were faculty at the most prestigious research universities in the country, operating within the normal structures of academic medicine and government-funded research.

Three categories from the committee's findings are documented here.

The Plutonium Injections. Between 1945 and 1947, eighteen patients — most terminally ill with cancer — were injected with plutonium without being told what they were receiving. The experiments were conducted at hospitals in California, Illinois, New York, and Tennessee. The researchers' objective was to study how the human body metabolizes plutonium — information useful for managing radiation exposure in workers at the nuclear weapons facilities that had produced the bombs used against Japan.

The patients were not weapons facility workers. They were hospital patients who had come for treatment of their underlying conditions. They were told the injections were part of their medical treatment. They were not told they were receiving plutonium. They were not told the injections were experimental. They were not told the injections served a military research purpose rather than a therapeutic one.

The committee found that the informed consent obtained — where any consent was obtained at all — did not meet even the minimal standards of the era, let alone the Nuremberg Code's standard of voluntary informed consent.

**The Cincinnati Experiments.* Between 1960 and 1971, researchers at Cincinnati General Hospital subjected 87 cancer patients to whole-body radiation in doses substantially higher than therapeutic levels. The experiments were funded by the Department of Defense. Their purpose, documented in the grant applications, was to study the effects of radiation on military personnel — specifically, to determine what levels of radiation exposure would temporarily incapacitate soldiers in a nuclear battlefield environment. The patients were acting, without their knowledge, as proxies for soldiers. Their cancer was being used as institutional cover for a military research program.

The patient population was, as the committee documented, predominantly poor and Black. The committee found that the consent procedures were inadequate and that the experimental nature of the radiation, its military purpose, and the doses involved were not disclosed to patients or their families.

Of the 87 patients subjected to the experiments, 8 died within sixty days of radiation — a rate the committee found significantly higher than expected. The committee concluded the evidence was insufficient to determine whether the radiation caused these deaths. It also concluded that the researchers had not adequately investigated the relationship between the radiation and the deaths.

**The Prison Experiments.* Between 1963 and 1973, researchers at Oregon State Penitentiary and Washington State Penitentiary irradiated the testicles of 67 inmates to study the effects of radiation on human fertility. The researchers were contracted by the Atomic Energy Commission. The inmates received small cash payments and signed consent forms.

The committee found that the consent forms did not adequately disclose the long-term risks of the procedure — including the possibility of chromosomal damage and testicular cancer. The committee also noted the fundamental ethical question of whether meaningful voluntary consent is possible in an institutional environment where the subject is under coercive confinement and where refusal may carry implicit costs to institutional status or privilege.

III. WHAT THE TWO PROGRAMS SHARE

Tuskegee and the radiation experiments were not related programs. They operated under different agencies, with different research objectives, in different institutional environments, across overlapping but not identical time periods. The researchers did not coordinate with each other. They did not share a stated ideology.

What they share is structural.

Both selected their experimental populations on the same logic: people whose objections were unlikely to be effective and whose suffering was unlikely to be attributed to the experiment. Black men in Macon County, Alabama, in 1932 and through 1972. Terminally ill cancer patients in 1945. Poor, predominantly Black patients at a city hospital in Cincinnati. Prison inmates in Oregon and Washington.

The verse that opens this chapter is from Proverbs 31. Its context is a king's mother instructing him in justice. The instruction is specific: open your mouth for people who cannot speak for themselves; defend people who cannot defend themselves. The verse names what justice requires. The two programs documented in this chapter name what justice's failure looks like when the institutions built to provide it become, instead, the mechanism of the harm.

Both programs were conducted by researchers who published their findings in peer-reviewed journals. Both were funded by government agencies. Both operated within the normal institutional structures of American science and medicine. Neither required secrecy to continue — Tuskegee's findings were in the published literature for forty years. What they required was the unspoken institutional assumption that the populations they used were available for use.

That assumption was not imported from Germany. It was not produced by Cold War emergency. It was the assumption that Chapter 1 documented at the ideological level and Chapter 2 documented at the institutional level: that some human bodies exist to be managed in the service of institutional goals, that their biological integrity is subject to institutional override when the institutional interest is sufficiently important, and that their objections can be safely ignored because the institutional power arrayed against them is sufficient to contain those objections.

The ideology was native. The programs proved it worked. The accountability was a formal apology, decades later, to the survivors who remained.

IV. NO PROSECUTIONS

The Advisory Committee's findings were delivered to President Clinton in October 1995. Clinton expressed regret on behalf of the government. He established a National Bioethics Advisory

Commission to develop guidance on human subjects research going forward. He did not order prosecutions. No researcher who had conducted the documented experiments was charged with a crime. No institution that had hosted them was sanctioned beyond the receipt of the government's formal regret.

The researchers who had irradiated prisoners in Oregon and Washington, the physicians who had injected patients with plutonium without disclosure, the Public Health Service officials who had watched syphilis kill dozens of men rather than end an observation study — they were not criminals in the eyes of the American legal system. They were researchers who had operated within the normal institutional culture of their era.

That is the most important finding the committee's work produced. Not that rogue actors had done terrible things. That an institutional culture had developed in which terrible things were normal — in which the populations documented above were routinely understood as available for use, in which the Nuremberg Code's "absolutely essential" standard of voluntary informed consent was a document about Germans and was not applied to what happened in American hospitals and prisons.

The committee concluded its report with a set of recommendations for reform of human subjects research oversight. The federal regulations governing research on human subjects — the Common Rule — had been in place since 1991. The committee recommended strengthening it. The regulations were amended. The institutional culture they were designed to constrain is the institutional culture documented across every chapter of this book.

The regulations are not the same thing as the culture.

PRIMARY SOURCES FOR THIS CHAPTER

Tuskegee:

- Advisory Committee on Human Radiation Experiments, *Final Report* (U.S. Government Printing Office, 1995). Available through the Department of Energy's OpenNet system at opennet.energy.gov. The committee reviewed the Tuskegee study in the context of its broader investigation of non-consensual government research.

- James H. Jones, *Bad Blood: The Tuskegee Syphilis Experiment* (Free Press, 1981; expanded 1993). The definitive documented history, drawing on PHS records, congressional investigation files, and interviews with surviving participants.

- The study's own published papers: Vonderlehr, R.A., et al., "Untreated Syphilis in the Male Negro," *Venereal Disease Information* 17 (1936); Rivers, E., et al., "Twenty Years of Followup Experience in a Long-Range Medical Study," *Public Health Reports* 68 (1953); Olansky, S., et al., "Untreated Syphilis in the Male Negro," *Journal of Chronic Diseases* 4 (1956). Available through the National Library of Medicine. These papers document the study in the researchers' own language across its full operation.

- "Tuskegee Syphilis Study: 1973 Ad Hoc Advisory Panel Report," available through the National Archives and cited in Jones's account. The panel's finding of "ethical unjustifiability."

- President Clinton's formal apology to surviving Tuskegee participants, May 16, 1997. Available through the Clinton Presidential Library and through the National Archives.

The Radiation Experiments:

- Advisory Committee on Human Radiation Experiments, *Final Report* (U.S. Government Printing Office, 1995). The primary source for all radiation experiment documentation in this chapter. Available in full at opennet.energy.gov. The report includes detailed findings on the plutonium injections (Chapter 5), the Cincinnati experiments (Chapter 8), and the prison experiments (Chapter 7), with primary source citations throughout.

- Eileen Welsome, *The Plutonium Files: America's Secret Medical Experiments in the Cold War* (Dial Press, 1999). Welsome won the Pulitzer Prize for investigative reporting for her original reporting on the plutonium experiments, which preceded and helped prompt the Clinton executive order establishing the advisory committee. Her book draws on documents obtained through FOIA.

- The original AEC grant applications and research reports for the Cincinnati experiments, referenced in the ACHRE Final Report and available through the Department of Energy OpenNet system.

The ACHRE Final Report is the foundational document for this chapter's radiation experiments content. It is a government document, produced by a government-appointed committee, drawing on government records. Its findings are not contested in any serious historical scholarship. The reader who wants to understand the scope and character of the radiation experiments is directed to the report itself — 925 pages, available online — and specifically to its executive summary, which presents the committee's principal findings in accessible form.

Chapter 6: The Suppression Architecture

COINTELPRO, Mass Surveillance, and the Management of Resistance

"Woe to those who decree iniquitous decrees, and the writers who keep writing oppression, to turn aside the needy from justice and to rob the poor of my people of their right."

— Isaiah 10:1–2

The programs documented in Chapters 4 and 5 shared a structural vulnerability.

The communities most likely to notice what was being done to them were the communities it was most directly being done to. Black Americans in the South knew what the Tuskegee study was — not in its details, not in its formal research design, but in the texture of lived experience with institutions that did not serve them. Native American communities on reservations knew what federal health programs had done to their women. The urban Black communities that had produced the Black Panther Party had direct, generational, embodied knowledge that American institutions were not structured for their protection.

These were also the communities with the most developed organizational capacity for political resistance. By the mid-1960s, the civil rights movement had demonstrated that organized political pressure could change law. The Black Panther Party had established free health clinics in communities systematically underserved by the medical system. The American Indian Movement was organizing to contest the federal sterilization programs that had continued into the 1970s, performing sterilizations on Native women — sometimes without informed consent, sometimes on minors — at Indian Health Service facilities. These organizations represented the specific threat the apparatus could not sustain: organized communities with legitimate grievances and the political capacity to make those grievances visible.

COINTELPRO addressed the vulnerability.

I. THE PROGRAM: DOCUMENTATION

The FBI's Counterintelligence Program — COINTELPRO — operated from 1956 to 1971. Its existence was not known to the public, to Congress, or to most of the government outside the FBI until March 8, 1971, when a group of activists burglarized the FBI's field office in Media, Pennsylvania, removed filing cabinets full of documents, and distributed what they found to newspapers across the country.

Most newspapers refused to publish what they received. The *Los Angeles Times*, the *New York Times*, and others declined, citing national security concerns at the FBI's request. The *Washington Post*, after its editor Ben Bradlee reviewed the documents and consulted the newspaper's lawyers, published. The documents entered the public record.

The subsequent investigation — the Church Committee, formally the United States Senate Select Committee to Study Governmental Operations with Respect to Intelligence Activities — produced the most comprehensive public accounting of COINTELPRO's scope and methods. The Church Committee's *Final Report, Books II and III*, published by the U.S. Government Printing Office in 1976, is available through the Senate archives and through the National Security Archive at George Washington University. Everything that follows is sourced from it and from the primary documents it reviewed.

The Church Committee found that COINTELPRO had targeted not only the organizations it publicly characterized as threats — the

Communist Party, various socialist organizations — but a much broader range of domestic political activity. The program had operated against: the NAACP, the Southern Christian Leadership Conference, the Student Nonviolent Coordinating Committee, the Black Panther Party, the American Indian Movement, the National Lawyers Guild, the Socialist Workers Party, and a range of antiwar organizations. It had also, the committee found, targeted specific individuals whose political activities the FBI considered threatening — most prominently, Martin Luther King Jr.

Forty-five of COINTELPRO's documented operations targeted the Black Panther Party alone.

II. THE METHODS

The Church Committee documented COINTELPRO's operational techniques in detail. They included:

Informant infiltration. The FBI placed informants within targeted organizations, often at senior levels. These informants provided intelligence on membership, plans, and internal conflicts. They also actively worked to disrupt the organizations from within — spreading disinformation, manufacturing conflicts between factions, providing information to law enforcement that led to arrests.

Fabricated documents. The FBI created and distributed forged letters, fake newspapers, and fabricated communications designed to produce internal conflict, damage leadership, and create the appearance of organizational betrayal. The Church Committee documented specific cases in which fabricated documents had contributed to violence — including, in the committee's assessment, contributing to conditions that led to the deaths of Black Panther members.

Anonymous letters and "poison pen" campaigns. The FBI sent anonymous letters to the employers, families, and associates of targeted individuals, alleging criminal activity, sexual misconduct, or political extremism, designed to destroy the individual's personal and professional life.

Coordination with local law enforcement. The FBI coordinated with local police departments to enable harassment, surveillance, and arrest of targeted individuals and organizations. The committee found that this coordination had, in some cases, facilitated violence against targeted organizations by police departments that the FBI knew were hostile.

The King letter. The Church Committee documented what the FBI had done to Martin Luther King Jr. with particular care, because what it documented was extraordinary. The FBI had maintained a file on King that ran to hundreds of thousands of pages. It had conducted intensive surveillance of his communications, his travels, and his personal life through illegal wiretaps and informants. After King was awarded the Nobel Peace Prize in October 1964, FBI Director J. Edgar Hoover escalated the operation.

In November 1964, the FBI sent King an anonymous letter — drafted in FBI offices — that referenced the surveillance material it had collected on his personal life and threatened to make this material public unless King took action "before your filthy, abnormal fraudulent self is bared to the nation." The letter concluded, in language the Church Committee quoted directly in its report: "There is but one way out for you. You better take it before your filthy, abnormal self is exposed to the nation. You are finished." A tape recording was enclosed as a threat.

The FBI's purpose, as the committee documented, was to induce King to commit suicide before he could receive the Nobel Prize. The letter was drafted by FBI officials. It was reviewed and approved in the chain of command. It was sent from a U.S. Post

Office.

The letter is in the congressional record. The Church Committee reproduced it.

No one who drafted, approved, or sent it was prosecuted.

III. THE SPECIFIC OVERLAP

The reader who has followed Chapters 4 and 5 carefully will notice an overlap that the primary sources establish but that is rarely named together.

The communities COINTELPRO concentrated its most intensive operations against — Black political organizations, indigenous rights organizations, the organized poor — were the same communities that had been concentrated in the experimental programs documented in Chapter 5.

Tuskegee ran from 1932 to 1972. COINTELPRO ran from 1956 to 1971. For fifteen years, the FBI's systematic political neutralization of Black organizational capacity and the Public Health Service's ongoing deliberate withholding of syphilis treatment from Black men in Alabama were running simultaneously. The communities most likely to organize effective resistance to the Tuskegee study's continuation — the communities with the direct experience, the moral authority, and the organizational capacity to demand accountability — were the communities COINTELPRO was simultaneously neutralizing.

The Indian Health Service's sterilization program for Native women — which the Government Accounting Office documented in 1976 as having sterilized between 25 and 50 percent of Native American women in some communities — ran in the same period as the American Indian Movement's organizing, which COINTELPRO targeted.

This book does not assert that COINTELPRO was designed specifically to protect Tuskegee or the IHS sterilization program. The primary sources do not establish that specific coordination. What they establish is the structural relationship: the experimental program and the suppression architecture shared a target. The communities most directly harmed by the former were the communities most directly neutralized by the latter. The coincidence of target, across programs that were not administratively coordinated, is itself a finding. The reader is invited to evaluate what it means.

Isaiah's indictment of those who "decree iniquitous decrees" and "rob the poor of my people of their right" is not addressed to criminals. It is addressed to administrators — to the writers of official documents, the decreers of official policy, the people with institutional authority and the institutional will to use it against the people least able to resist it. The verse names a specific form of institutional evil: the formal, bureaucratic, documented, systematically organized abuse of the power that was supposed to protect.

That is what both programs documented in this chapter were.

IV. THE SCALE THAT FOLLOWED: SNOWDEN

Senator Frank Church, who chaired the committee that documented COINTELPRO, made an observation in 1975 about the surveillance capabilities the NSA had already developed. He said: "That capability at any time could be turned around on the American people, and no American would have any privacy left, such is the capability to monitor everything — telephone conversations, telegrams, it doesn't matter. There would be no place to hide."

He made that observation thirty-eight years before Edward

Snowden walked out of an NSA facility in Hawaii with four laptops containing the documentation of what had been built.

Glenn Greenwald's *No Place to Hide* (Metropolitan Books, 2014), based directly on the documents Snowden provided, documented the programs Church had warned about: PRISM, which accessed communications data directly from the servers of major technology companies including Google, Apple, Facebook, and Microsoft; XKeyscore, a search tool capable of querying the full content of intercepted internet traffic; MUSCULAR, which intercepted data flowing between Google and Yahoo data centers overseas; and Section 215 bulk metadata collection, which gathered the call records of essentially every American with a phone.

The documents themselves — not Greenwald's account of them, the documents — are in the public record, published by *The Guardian*, *The Washington Post*, and other outlets that received them from Snowden. They are archived at theintercept.com. The reader who wants to see what population-scale surveillance looks like in operational documentation is directed there.

The Church Committee had created oversight structures after COINTELPRO was exposed: the Foreign Intelligence Surveillance Court, the requirement for judicial approval of domestic wiretaps, the prohibition on assassination of foreign leaders. The post-September 11 emergency framework — the PATRIOT Act, the executive orders authorizing the NSA programs Snowden documented — was built to operate around those oversight structures rather than within them. The legal architecture of emergency authorization, familiar from every previous chapter of this book, performed the same function here that it performed in MKUltra, in the mRNA vaccine deployment, in the hospital protocols of 2020: it removed the accountability structures that had been created in response to previous abuses and replaced them with the institutional judgment of the agencies conducting the new programs.

The scale changed. The structure did not.

V. THE CLOSE OF PART TWO

Part Two of this book is complete.

Chapter 3 documented the transfer of the experimental ideology from Nazi Germany to American soil. Chapter 4 documented how that ideology operated in practice: non-consenting human beings subjected to pharmacological assault and psychological torture in a program that ran for twenty years in eighty institutions. Chapter 5 documented that the ideology required no import — it was already native, operating in programs that predated Paperclip and continued long after it. Chapter 6 has documented the suppression architecture built around those programs: the systematic neutralization of the organizational capacity of the communities most directly harmed, scaled from informant networks to population-level surveillance.

The apparatus now has its experimental methodology, its proven tolerance for institutional accountability, its suppression architecture, and its scale.

Part Three documents how it captured the institutions that remained — the regulatory agencies, the food system, the childhood health infrastructure, the enforcement network that kept the captured inside and the resistant neutralized. By the end of Part Three, the pen is complete.

PRIMARY SOURCES FOR THIS CHAPTER

COINTELPRO:

- United States Senate Select Committee to Study Governmental Operations with Respect to Intelligence Activities (Church Committee), *Final Report, Books II and III* (U.S. Government Printing Office, 1976). Available through the Senate Historical Office and at the National Security Archive (nsarchive.gwu.edu). Book II covers intelligence activities and civil rights; Book III covers domestic intelligence programs including COINTELPRO. The FBI letter to King is reproduced in Book III.

- Betty Medsger, *The Burglary: The Discovery of J. Edgar Hoover's Secret FBI* (Knopf, 2014). The authoritative account of the Media, Pennsylvania break-in, drawing on the documents themselves and on decades of reporting, including interviews with the activists who conducted the burglary. The book documents how COINTELPRO came to public light.

- Ward Churchill and Jim Vander Wall, *The COINTELPRO Papers: Documents from the FBI's Secret Wars Against Dissent in the United States* (South End Press, 1990; updated 2002). Compiles primary COINTELPRO documents with contextual analysis.

- Government Accountability Office, "Investigation of Allegations Concerning Indian Health Service," report B-164031(5), November 1976. The GAO's own investigation of the Indian Health Service sterilization program, documented at gao.gov.

Snowden and Mass Surveillance:

- Glenn Greenwald, *No Place to Hide: Edward Snowden, the NSA, and the U.S. Surveillance State* (Metropolitan Books, 2014). Documents the NSA programs including PRISM, XKeyscore, MUSCULAR, and Section 215 collection, drawing directly on the documents Snowden provided.

- The Intercept, Snowden documents archive — theintercept.com.

The primary document archive for NSA surveillance programs revealed by Snowden. The documents themselves are available for direct review.

- Senator Frank Church, NBC's *Meet the Press*, August 17, 1975. Church's warning about NSA surveillance capabilities is documented in multiple accounts of the Church Committee period and is quoted in Greenwald's account with citation.

- Foreign Intelligence Surveillance Act (1978), Public Law 95-511. The legislative response to the Church Committee, available at congress.gov. Provides the legal context for understanding what the post-9/11 surveillance architecture was built to circumvent.

The Church Committee Final Report is, like the ACHRE Report, a government document produced by a government-appointed body, drawing on government records, finding government wrongdoing. Its findings are not contested in any serious historical scholarship. The reader who doubts this chapter's account of COINTELPRO is invited to read the primary congressional record — Books II and III of the Final Report — directly. The FBI letter to Martin Luther King is in the congressional record. The reader can verify it.

Chapter 7: The Regulatory Revolving Door

FDA, CDC, USDA, EPA — By Name, Position, and Date

"Woe to those who call evil good and good evil, who put darkness for light and light for darkness, who put bitter for sweet and sweet for bitter."

— Isaiah 5:20

There is a word for what happens when the agency built to protect the public from an industry becomes the agency that protects that industry from the public. The word is capture. It is used in academic literature on regulatory economics, in congressional testimony, in peer-reviewed public health journals. It is not a conspiracy theory. It is a documented structural phenomenon with a documented mechanism, documented personnel, and documented consequences measured in human lives.

This chapter documents the capture of the Food and Drug Administration — the federal agency whose stated mission is to protect and promote public health by ensuring the safety and efficacy of the drugs, biologics, and medical devices that Americans consume. It documents the specific mechanism by which that capture was accomplished: the systematic movement of personnel between the regulator and the regulated, in both directions, across decades, in patterns that are now quantified in peer-reviewed literature and confirmed in the records of the institutions themselves.

It uses names. It uses dates. It uses the documented record.

Because the capture is not a theory. It is a career trajectory. And career trajectories are in the public record.

I. THE MECHANISM: HOW THE DOOR WAS BUILT

The modern pharmaceutical regulatory apparatus runs on a funding model that would strike any disinterested observer as structurally indefensible: the industry that the FDA regulates pays, directly, for the salaries of the people who regulate it.

This arrangement has a name and a date. The Prescription Drug User Fee Act — PDUFA — was passed by Congress in 1992 and signed into law by President George H.W. Bush. It authorized the FDA to collect fees from pharmaceutical manufacturers at the time of new drug applications, with those funds designated specifically for the drug review process. In fiscal year 1993, the FDA collected $66 million in industry user fees. By 2018, that figure had grown to over $900 million annually. By 2026, industry user fees account for approximately 51% of the FDA's total program budget — and approximately 80% of the salaries of the drug application reviewers themselves.

Read that again: the people whose job is to determine whether a pharmaceutical company's drug is safe enough to sell to the American public have approximately 80% of their salaries paid by the pharmaceutical industry.

The PDUFA legislation came with performance benchmarks — targets for how quickly the FDA must complete its drug reviews. Miss the benchmark, and the industry can object to the fee arrangement at the next reauthorization cycle, which occurs every five years. The pressure is structural and continuous: approve drugs faster, or risk the funding that pays for the staff who approve the drugs. A peer-reviewed analysis published in the medical literature found that drugs approved after the passage of PDUFA were more likely to be subsequently withdrawn for safety reasons than drugs approved before it. The funding model, in other words, demonstrably accelerated approvals at the expense of safety — and the acceleration is documented in the outcomes.

This is the first layer of capture: financial. The FDA is institutionally dependent on the continued goodwill of the industry it nominally regulates.

The second layer is personnel. And this is where the names enter.

II. THE NUMBERS: WHAT THE RESEARCH ESTABLISHED

In 2016, Dr. Vinay Prasad and his colleague published a study in *The BMJ* — one of the world's most prestigious peer-reviewed medical journals — that for the first time quantified what had previously been known only anecdotally. They examined the job histories of 55 FDA staff members who had conducted drug reviews in the hematology-oncology field over a nine-year period.

Their finding: more than a quarter of the FDA employees who approved cancer and hematology drugs from 2001 through 2010 subsequently left the agency to work or consult for the pharmaceutical industry — and in a significant number of cases, for the specific companies whose drugs they had previously reviewed.

A follow-up analysis by *Science* magazine found the pattern holding across the agency: FDA staffers who approved drugs went on to work for the makers of those same drugs at rates that raised consistent conflict-of-interest questions. The companies hiring them were not paying for their general expertise. They were paying for their institutional knowledge, their relationships, and their understanding of exactly how to navigate the approval process they had just administered from the other side.

An independent financial study published in 2023 on the Social Science Research Network quantified the downstream effect: when pharmaceutical companies hire former FDA employees, their drug approval rates increase. When the former FDA employee held a higher-ranked executive position, the effect is more pronounced. The study found this effect was statistically robust across multiple controls.

The revolving door, in other words, is not merely a reputational problem. It produces measurable, documented outcomes. Hiring the right former FDA official increases a pharmaceutical company's probability of approval. This is the market clearing price for regulatory capture — and it is paid, openly, in the employment records of the people involved.

III. THE NAMES: DOCUMENTED CASES

Dr. Curtis Wright and OxyContin

The most catastrophic single drug approval in American history has a face, a name, and a career trajectory.

In December 1995, the FDA approved OxyContin — Purdue Pharma's extended-release oxycodone formulation — for the treatment of moderate to severe pain. The approval was based on clinical trials that had not been specifically designed to assess the drug's abuse potential. The lead medical reviewer responsible for the approval was Dr. Curtis Wright IV, then acting director of the FDA division responsible for approving the drug: the Division of Anesthetic, Critical Care, and Addiction Drug Products.

The OxyContin label that Wright's division approved contained a crucial sentence: "Delayed absorption, as provided by OxyContin tablets, is believed to reduce the abuse liability of the drug." This sentence — phrased deliberately as belief rather than established fact, without the clinical evidence that would normally be required for such a claim — became the central marketing weapon Purdue deployed to expand OxyContin's prescription base from severe cancer pain to moderate chronic pain conditions affecting tens of millions of Americans.

The sentence had no scientific basis. Internal Purdue documents produced in subsequent litigation showed the company knew it. A 2006 Department of Justice memorandum written by deputy chief of the DOJ fraud section Kirk Orgosky — which documented a recommendation to indict Purdue Pharma for mail fraud, wire fraud, and money laundering — noted that Purdue had "traveled to the FDA's location in Rockland, Maryland in January and February of 1995 and rented a room nearby," and that it was highly likely Wright had spent multiple days helping Purdue write the safety and efficacy studies for OxyContin's application. Purdue Pharma officials later claimed the critical abuse-liability sentence was added "at FDA's suggestion." Wright, in a sworn deposition, acknowledged he "might" have written it.

Two years after approving OxyContin, Wright left the FDA and took a position at Purdue Pharma. His first-year compensation package was $379,000 — approximately three times his government salary. He was not the only one. The second principal medical reviewer who originally approved the OxyContin application, Dr. Douglas Kramer, also subsequently went to work for Purdue.

The two FDA officials most directly responsible for the approval that launched the opioid epidemic both went to work for the company whose drug they had approved.

The American Journal of Medicine Ethics — a publication of the American Medical Association — stated this plainly in a 2020 analysis: "The 2 principal FDA reviewers who originally approved Purdue's oxycodone application both took positions at Purdue after leaving the agency." The FDA, the analysis noted, "has never been held to account for its improper handling of the opioid crisis."

The opioid crisis has killed more than 800,000 Americans since 1999. By 2013 — the year that, by one measure, represented the peak of prescription opioid abuse — enough opioids were prescribed in the United States to provide every American adult with a full bottle of pills. The CDC calls this the "first wave" of the opioid epidemic. Purdue Pharma earned over $30 billion from OxyContin sales. In 2007, it pleaded guilty to federal charges of misbranding, paying $600 million in fines. In 2020, it pleaded guilty again and paid $8 billion. The Sackler family, which owned Purdue, has paid billions in civil settlements while admitting no personal wrongdoing.

The FDA has never conducted a public root-cause analysis of its own role in the approval.

Scott Gottlieb and Pfizer

On March 5, 2019, FDA Commissioner Scott Gottlieb announced his resignation from the agency he had led for nearly two years. He stated that he wanted to spend more time with his family.

On June 27, 2019 — 85 days after leaving the FDA — Gottlieb was announced as a member of Pfizer's board of directors. A seat on the Pfizer board paid more than $330,000 annually in cash and company stock. He was also appointed to the board's Regulatory and Compliance Committee and its Science and Technology Committee.

The appointment drew immediate response from across the political spectrum. Senator Elizabeth Warren wrote to Gottlieb on July 1, 2019: "This kind of revolving door influence-peddling smacks of corruption, and makes the American people rightfully cynical and distrustful." Public Citizen's Dr. Sidney Wolfe observed: "Philosophically, he's returning to the ecosystem where he's most comfortable. And he'll get paid very well for it."

The timing had a specific quality. A July 3 story in the *Milwaukee Journal Sentinel* reported that the FDA under Gottlieb, just weeks before his resignation, had taken less aggressive regulatory action than European regulators on safety concerns about Pfizer's drug tofacitinib (Xeljanz). University of Minnesota bioethicist Dr. Carl Elliott told the paper: "It sounds like a reward for a job well done."

Gottlieb's prior career had run through the pharmaceutical industry before his FDA appointment — he was a partner at venture capital firm New Enterprise Associates and had served on the boards of multiple pharmaceutical companies before taking the FDA role, from which he had been required to recuse himself on matters involving those companies. He returned to all of it, and added Pfizer, within months of his departure.

The Wikipedia entry for Scott Gottlieb, available in the public record, documents his current positions: member of the board of directors of Pfizer, Inc.; member of the board of directors of UnitedHealth Group; Chairman of the board of gene sequencing company Illumina. He is also a regular contributor to CNBC and CBS News, where he is identified as a former FDA commissioner offering expert opinion on pharmaceutical and public health matters — including, during the Covid period, on the vaccine products of the company whose board he sat on.

The Quantified Pattern

The Wright and Gottlieb cases are not anomalies. They are documented instances of a quantified pattern.

The Stanford Law Review published a 2023 analysis — "FDA's Revolving Door: Reckoning and Reform" — that conducted a scoping review of the revolving door specifically at the FDA. It found that 11 of 16 FDA medical examiners identified in a *Science* magazine study took post-government employment with companies they had formerly regulated. It documented the

Aduhelm (aducanumab) and Exondys 51 (eteplirsen) approval controversies — both involving "atypical associations between FDA regulators and pharmaceutical company sponsors" and "fierce internal disputes over the adequacy of the evidence." It identified the revolving door as "one persistent source of undue influence that overshadows the discharge of FDA regulators' duties to the public."

The *Science* magazine investigation that produced the underlying data — published in 2018 — found that FDA staffers who managed successful drug reviews were specifically and disproportionately targeted for recruitment by the companies whose drugs they had approved. The companies were not hiring for general pharmaceutical expertise. They were hiring the specific people who knew the specific drugs from inside the approval process. The value of the hire was the institutional knowledge plus, critically, the relationship — the personal knowledge of the people still inside the agency who would handle the next application.

At the time of the current writing, former FDA Commissioner Scott Gottlieb has estimated that as many as 600 drug reviewers have recused themselves from approval processes because they are simultaneously interviewing with pharmaceutical companies. Six hundred active FDA drug reviewers, at this moment, are in conversations with the companies whose drugs they are supposed to be evaluating with independence.

This is not a revolving door. It is a standing opening.

IV. THE STRUCTURAL CAPTURE: PDUFA AND ITS CONSEQUENCES

The individual career moves documented above occur within a structural context that makes them not aberrations but rational responses to institutional incentives. Understanding the structure is essential because the structure is what the book is about — not individual corruption but systemic capture that produces institutional behavior independent of the intentions of any individual participant.

PDUFA — the Prescription Drug User Fee Act — was not designed to corrupt the FDA. It was designed to solve a genuine problem: the FDA in the 1980s had a backlog of drug applications averaging 29 months to review, underfunded by a Congress that had not increased its appropriations. The pharmaceutical industry, which lost an estimated $10 million per month for each month of review delay, had obvious incentives to see reviews accelerated. User fees were the solution both sides could accept.

What the 1992 arrangement created, however, was a structural relationship in which the FDA's budget, its performance benchmarks, and its five-year reauthorization cycle are all negotiated with the industry it regulates. The PDUFA reauthorization process involves, according to the peer-reviewed analysis in *Academic Emergency Medicine*, more than 100 meetings between FDA and industry representatives to negotiate the terms of the next five-year cycle. The industry negotiates the performance goals to which the FDA will be held. The FDA agrees to those goals as the condition of continued funding.

The peer-reviewed literature on this relationship is unambiguous in its conclusions. A 2018 analysis in *Therapeutic Innovation and Regulatory Science* found that "drugs approved by the FDA after the passage of PDUFA were more likely to be withdrawn for safety reasons" than drugs approved before it. A 2022 analysis in *Academic Emergency Medicine* concluded that "the majority of policy changes enacted through PDUFA legislation have favored industry through decreasing regulatory standards, shortening approval times, and increasing industry involvement in FDA decision-making."

A more direct statement is difficult to find in peer-reviewed literature. Decreased regulatory standards. Shorter approval times. Increased industry involvement in FDA decision-making. These are not the outputs of an agency protecting the public. They are the outputs of a captured agency.

V. THE OPIOID CRISIS AS CASE STUDY IN COMPLETED CAPTURE

The opioid epidemic is the clearest documented demonstration of what a captured FDA produces.

The timeline is in the congressional record, in court documents produced in litigation against Purdue Pharma and other opioid manufacturers, and in the investigative record assembled by journalists, investigators, and the plaintiffs' attorneys who sued nearly every opioid manufacturer and distributor in the United States.

1995: OxyContin approved on the basis of clinical trials not designed to assess abuse potential, with an unsupported abuse-liability claim written into the label. The lead reviewer goes to work for Purdue two years later at triple his government salary.

1996–2000: OxyContin prescriptions for musculoskeletal pain — a use far beyond the severe cancer pain for which the drug's clinical evidence existed — increase twentyfold. Purdue's marketing budget is documented in internal records produced in litigation.

2001: FDA convenes an advisory committee to consider whether opioid labels should be narrowed to prohibit marketing for common chronic pain conditions. Eight of the ten outside experts on the committee have documented financial ties to pharmaceutical companies, including Purdue. The committee advises against narrowing the indication.

2001: FDA approves an updated OxyContin label expanding its approved use to around-the-clock pain management of an extended duration. Purdue's internal documents, produced in litigation and reported by Marketplace News which obtained them under court order, record the company's reaction: "The action by the FDA has created enormous opportunities." Sales triple.

2007: Purdue Pharma and three executives plead guilty to federal charges of misbranding OxyContin with intent to defraud and mislead, paying $600 million in fines. No senior executive goes to prison. The company continues selling OxyContin.

2019: Purdue Pharma files for bankruptcy. The Sackler family negotiates a settlement in which they pay billions of dollars to states, tribes, and municipalities while admitting no personal wrongdoing and retaining a substantial portion of their fortune.

2020: Purdue pleads guilty again to additional federal criminal charges related to its marketing of OxyContin, paying $8.3 billion in total fines and forfeitures.

From 1999 through 2021, approximately 645,000 Americans died from an overdose involving any opioid — prescription or illicit. The CDC documents this as having occurred in three waves: the first wave driven by prescription opioids; the second by heroin, as users whose prescription opioid supply was cut off turned to the street; the third by illicitly manufactured fentanyl, as the market adapted to enforcement pressure on prescription opioids.

The first wave was ignited by a single FDA approval in 1995, made by a reviewer who subsequently went to work for the company he approved, writing into the label language the company needed and that the science did not support.

The FDA has never conducted a public accounting of its role in any of these waves.

VI. THE ADVISORY COMMITTEE PROBLEM

The Curtis Wright and Scott Gottlieb cases are what happens at the top of the revolving door. But the capture operates at every level of the agency's decision-making structure, including its advisory committees — the panels of outside experts the FDA convenes to evaluate evidence and make recommendations on specific drug approvals.

The 2001 OxyContin label expansion advisory committee — eight of ten members with pharma financial ties — was not an anomaly. It was a consistent feature of how the FDA's advisory process operates.

A 2004 study in *JAMA* found that 28% of FDA advisory committee members had conflicts of interest that would have disqualified them from the panel under the agency's own rules — but that the FDA routinely granted waivers to allow conflicted experts to participate. A 2009 study in *PLOS Medicine* found that industry-funded members of FDA advisory committees voted to approve drugs at higher rates than non-conflicted members.

The FDA's own rules required disclosure of conflicts and, in some cases, recusal. The rules were routinely waived. The waivers were granted by the FDA. The agency that the advisory committees were supposed to provide independent expert input to was the same agency deciding which conflicted experts could serve on those committees.

The circularity is complete.

VII. THE FUNDING STRUCTURE BEYOND PDUFA

PDUFA is the most visible mechanism of pharmaceutical capture, but it operates alongside others that compound the structural problem.

The CDC Foundation — a nonprofit established by Congress in 1992 to support the CDC's public health mission — accepts direct donations from pharmaceutical companies, medical device manufacturers, and other industries regulated by the agencies in the CDC's orbit. The Foundation's donor list, available through its published annual reports, includes Pfizer, Johnson and Johnson, Merck, Abbott, and other companies with direct financial interests in the CDC's guidance, recommendations, and policy positions.

The FDA's own foundation, the Reagan-Udall Foundation, accepts industry funding for research projects and public health initiatives. Its board has included representatives from the pharmaceutical industry.

The revolving door at the CDC runs parallel to the one at the FDA: named former CDC officials move to pharmaceutical companies, consulting firms that serve pharmaceutical companies, and the pharmaceutical industry's lobbying apparatus in patterns documented by Kaiser Health News and others who have tracked the flows.

The cumulative effect is an agency that is funded by, staffed by, and surrounded by the industry it is supposed to regulate — at every level, from the staff reviewer to the commissioner, from the advisory committee member to the foundation board.

VIII. WHAT THE CAPTURE PRODUCES

The opioid crisis is the most lethal demonstration of completed capture. It is not the only one.

The Aduhelm (aducanumab) approval in 2021 — the controversial Alzheimer's drug approved by the FDA over the objections of its own advisory committee, all but one of whose members recommended against approval, with ten members subsequently resigning in protest — demonstrated the same pattern at the level of the agency's leadership. The FDA approved Aduhelm using an accelerated pathway typically reserved for drugs with clear evidence of clinical benefit. The agency's own advisory committee had found the clinical trial data insufficient to support approval. Three members of Congress formally called for an investigation. The Department of Health and Human Services Office of Inspector General opened a formal investigation into the FDA's interactions with the drug's manufacturer, Biogen, during the review process. CMS ultimately decided that Medicare would only cover Aduhelm for patients enrolled in clinical trials — effectively limiting its use to the research setting the original approval process should have confined it to.

The Exondys 51 (eteplirsen) approval in 2016 — a Duchenne muscular dystrophy treatment approved over the explicit objection of the FDA's own statistical reviewers and advisory committee — involved documented internal dissent that was overridden by senior FDA leadership. The drug's efficacy was based on a surrogate endpoint so weakly correlated with clinical benefit that the agency's own experts called it insufficient. The approval nonetheless proceeded. The manufacturer, Sarepta Therapeutics, had been an active participant in the PDUFA reauthorization negotiations.

In both cases: internal dissent. External advisory committee objection. Approval over objection. No accountability.

The Stanford Law Review analysis puts the institutional conclusion plainly: the revolving door creates "an anticipated return to industry, which may lead officials to favor industry's interests over the public's during their tenure at the agency, in hopes of securing favorable employment after their government service."

This is the mechanism of capture stated in academic language. Translated: while they are at the FDA, officials favor the industry because they are already planning to work for it.

IX. THE LONG CONSEQUENCE

The pharmaceutical capture documented in this chapter produced the opioid epidemic. It produced the Aduhelm approval. It produced the Exondys approval. It produced, as Chapter 13 will document, the Emergency Use Authorization framework that deployed a novel vaccine technology at global scale without the long-term safety data that the capture had systematically made inconvenient to require.

These outcomes share a structure: the agency built to protect the public made decisions that protected the industry at the public's expense. The decisions were made by people who had come from the industry or were planning to return to it. The funding that paid their salaries came from the industry. The performance benchmarks they were judged against were negotiated with the industry. The advisory committees they convened included members paid by the industry.

The capture is structural, sustained, and documented in the primary sources this chapter has cited. It does not require a secret meeting or a deliberate conspiracy. It requires only the institutional architecture that PDUFA established and three decades of personnel decisions made rationally within that architecture.

By the time the Covid period arrived, the FDA was not an independent regulator. It was a dependent one. What a dependent regulator does when a crisis arrives and the industry it depends on presents a solution is documented in Chapter 13.

But before that, the chapter requires one observation that the academic literature makes carefully and that this book will make plainly:

The FDA captured by the pharmaceutical industry is not the same as an FDA that failed. A failed agency is one that tried to protect the public and fell short. The captured FDA is one that succeeded — at protecting the industry. By every metric the industry would use to measure its performance: faster approvals, more approvals, fewer regulatory obstacles, compliant advisory panels, sympathetic commissioners who understood that their next position depended on how well they managed the relationship during their current one.

The FDA has not failed. It has been very, very successful.

At the wrong job.

PRIMARY SOURCES FOR THIS CHAPTER

Legislation and Government Records:

- Prescription Drug User Fee Act of 1992, Public Law 102-571. Full text at congress.gov. The foundational document establishing the industry funding relationship.

- PDUFA reauthorization legislation — PDUFA II through VII — available at congress.gov. Documents the expansion of industry funding and performance goal negotiation across three decades.

- Congressional Research Service, "FDA Human Medical Product User Fee Programs" and "Prescription Drug User Fees," available at congress.gov/crs-products. Confirms the 51% budget share and 80% drug reviewer salary figure.

- HHS ASPE Issue Brief on FDA User Fees, available at aspe.hhs.gov. Confirms user fees account for 66% of the human drugs budget.

Peer-Reviewed Literature:

- Prasad, V., and S. Mailankody. "Research and development spending to bring a single cancer drug to market and revenues after approval." *JAMA Internal Medicine*, 2017. Documents the financial mechanics of pharmaceutical drug development and FDA approval.

- Karas, L. "FDA's Revolving Door: Reckoning and Reform." *Stanford Law & Policy Review*, 2023. The comprehensive academic analysis of the revolving door mechanism at the FDA. Available through Stanford Law School at law.stanford.edu.

- Analysis in *Academic Emergency Medicine* (2022) confirming PDUFA's effect on decreasing regulatory standards, shortening approval times, and increasing industry involvement in FDA decision-making.

- Roudini, S. "Unlocking the Revolving Door: How FDA-Firm Relationships Affect Drug Approval Rates and Innovation in the Pharmaceutical Industry." SSRN, 2023. Documents the approval rate increase following revolving door hires.

- "How FDA Failures Contributed to the Opioid Crisis." *Journal of Ethics*, American Medical Association, August 2020. Documents the Curtis Wright and Douglas Kramer post-FDA employment at Purdue. Available at journalofethics.ama-assn.org.

Investigative Journalism Based on Primary Documents:

- Marketplace News investigation into OxyContin's FDA approval, 2017. Obtained FDA-Purdue meeting minutes under court order. Documents the 2001 label expansion and Purdue's internal response.

- *Science* magazine investigation, "FDA's revolving door: Companies often hire agency staffers who managed their successful drug reviews," July 2018.

- Kaiser Health News analysis, "Big Pharma greets hundreds of ex-federal workers at the 'revolving door,'" 2018. Documents the congressional revolving door alongside the agency one.

- Public Citizen, "Outrage of the Month: Revolving Door to FDA Commissioner's Office Sows Distrust in Agency," October 2019. Documents the Gottlieb-Pfizer timeline.

Court Records and Litigation Documents:

- Department of Justice memorandum by Kirk Orgosky (2006) recommending indictment of Purdue Pharma. Documents Wright's involvement in writing OxyContin clinical studies.

- Purdue Pharma bankruptcy proceedings — the financial record of OxyContin's revenue and the settlement amounts.

- Purdue Pharma guilty pleas: 2007 (misbranding with intent to defraud, $600 million) and 2020 ($8.3 billion).

Named Personnel Records:

- Dr. Curtis Wright: FDA Division of Anesthetic, Critical Care, and Addiction Drug Products. OxyContin approval 1995. Purdue Pharma executive director of medical research, 1998. First-year compensation $379,000. Documented in sworn deposition testimony, court records, and Patrick Radden Keefe, *Empire of Pain* (Doubleday, 2021).

- Dr. Scott Gottlieb: FDA Commissioner May 2017–April 2019. Pfizer board member from June 2019. Board compensation exceeding $330,000 annually. Documented in Pfizer's own public announcement (June 27, 2019), CNBC, and all major financial news outlets. Senator Warren's letter (July 1, 2019) available at warren.senate.gov.

All sources in this chapter are primary documents, official records, peer-reviewed literature, or reporting directly based on court-ordered document releases. The reader is encouraged to verify independently. The sources are in the public record.

Chapter 8: The Food System

Seed Monopolies, Chemical Agriculture, and the Engineering of Chronic Illness

"And God said, Behold, I have given you every plant yielding seed that is on the face of all the earth, and every tree with seed in its fruit. You shall have them for food."

— Genesis 1:29

The food was given. It belonged to everyone who lived on the earth. The seeds belonged to every farmer who planted them, saved them, and passed them to the next generation. The soil belonged to the communities that cultivated it. The knowledge of what nourished the human body accumulated over millennia of observation, practice, and tradition, belonging to no corporation and requiring no patent.

That was the condition the apparatus set out to change.

The food system capture documented in this chapter did not happen in a single act of institutional seizure. It happened in layers, across decades, through the same mechanisms documented in Chapter 7 — the use of science as a commercial instrument, the capture of regulatory bodies, the weaponization of patent law — applied not to medicine but to agriculture and nutrition. The result is a food supply in which the seeds that produce most of what Americans eat are owned by a handful of corporations, saturated with chemicals whose cancer links were known internally while being publicly denied, and processed in ways specifically engineered to override the human body's natural satiety mechanisms and produce chronic illness that generates pharmaceutical revenue.

This is not an interpretation of the evidence. It is the evidence. And because the companies involved in this capture made the mistake of putting it in writing, the internal documents exist — in court records, in FOIA archives, in the published analyses of researchers who obtained them.

This chapter documents what those documents show.

I. THE DIETARY SCIENCE CAPTURE: HOW THE SUGAR INDUSTRY REWROTE NUTRITIONAL POLICY

Before the seed monopolies. Before Roundup. Before the food pyramid. There was a decision made in the 1960s by a trade organization representing the sugar industry that would shape American dietary policy — and American health — for the next sixty years.

The decision was documented in internal industry records found in public archives and analyzed by researchers at the University of California San Francisco. Their findings were published on September 12, 2016, in *JAMA Internal Medicine* — one of the most prestigious peer-reviewed medical journals in the United States. The paper was titled "Sugar Industry and Coronary Heart Disease Research: A Historical Analysis of Internal Industry Documents." Its authors were Cristin E. Kearns, Laura A. Schmidt, and Stanton A. Glantz.

What Kearns, Schmidt, and Glantz found in more than 340 documents totaling 1,582 pages of correspondence between the Sugar Research Foundation and Harvard University researchers was this:

In the 1950s, early evidence began linking sugar consumption to elevated blood cholesterol and triglyceride levels — both recognized risk factors for coronary heart disease. Simultaneously, a competing hypothesis linked dietary fat to heart disease. The sugar industry — whose internal documents showed it had recognized as early as 1954 that if Americans adopted low-fat diets, per-capita sugar consumption would increase by more than one-third — had a direct financial interest in the fat hypothesis winning.

In 1965, the Sugar Research Foundation commissioned Project 226: a literature review to be written by Harvard University nutrition scientists D. Mark Hegsted and Fredrick Stare. The SRF set the review's objective, contributed articles for inclusion, and received drafts throughout the process. The industry paid the Harvard scientists the equivalent of $50,000 in 2016 dollars. The SRF's funding of the review and its role in shaping its contents were not disclosed in the final publication.

The review appeared in the *New England Journal of Medicine* in 1967. It singled out fat and cholesterol as the primary dietary causes of coronary heart disease. It downplayed the evidence linking sugar consumption to the same diseases. It argued that blood cholesterol levels were the only significant risk factor for coronary heart disease — a framing that conveniently made the high sugar content of the American diet appear less hazardous.

The paper was not one study among many. It became the foundational reference that shaped the direction of nutritional science for a generation. The fat-versus-carbohydrate debate in nutrition was decided — not by the weight of the evidence, but by an undisclosed industry commission to Harvard scientists.

D. Mark Hegsted, one of the two principal authors of the industry-funded review, later became administrator of the USDA's Office of Nutrition — the official most directly responsible for translating nutritional science into federal dietary guidelines. In 1980, Hegsted's office produced the first *Dietary Guidelines for Americans*.

The first *Dietary Guidelines for Americans* recommended reducing dietary fat and increasing carbohydrate consumption. The food pyramid that followed placed grains at its base, recommending six to eleven servings daily. The low-fat era — which produced the explosion of low-fat processed foods that replaced natural fats with refined carbohydrates and added sugars — was built on nutritional science that the internal documents of the sugar industry show was purchased, directed, and shaped to produce a predetermined conclusion.

The JAMA Internal Medicine paper's senior author, Dr. Stanton Glantz of UCSF, summarized the finding in terms borrowed from the tobacco industry's own internal documentation: "As the saying goes, he who pays the piper calls the tune."

The piper, in this case, played the tune that the American food industry needed. And the American public danced to it for sixty years, while rates of obesity, type 2 diabetes, and metabolic syndrome climbed in direct correlation with the carbohydrate-heavy dietary recommendations the purchased science had produced.

In the 2020-2025 edition of the *Dietary Guidelines for Americans*, the U.S. federal government rejected the advice of its own expert scientific advisory panel to set lower targets for added sugar consumption. The Sugar Research Foundation's investment in Project 226, made in 1965, was still paying returns.

II. THE CHEMICAL CAPTURE: GLYPHOSATE, THE MONSANTO PAPERS, AND THE EPA

The same playbook that the sugar industry used on nutritional science — purchase the research, shape the conclusions, suppress the contradictory findings, capture the regulatory determination — was deployed by Monsanto over the following three decades on behalf of its flagship herbicide, glyphosate, the active ingredient in Roundup.

Roundup became the most widely used herbicide in human history. It was used on farms, in gardens, on schoolyards, on roadsides. By the time the litigation began that would ultimately force the release of Monsanto's internal documents, glyphosate was present in the food supply, in drinking water, in the urine of a significant fraction of the American population, and in the bodies of people who had never intentionally used it.

In 2015, the World Health Organization's International Agency for Research on Cancer — the IARC, the foremost independent cancer research authority in the world — classified glyphosate as a probable human carcinogen, Group 2A. The cancer most strongly associated with glyphosate exposure in the epidemiological literature was non-Hodgkin lymphoma.

What happened next is documented in millions of pages of internal Monsanto documents produced under court order as part of the Roundup cancer litigation — a body of evidence now known as the Monsanto Papers, archived by the litigation firm Wisner Baum and by the investigative organization U.S. Right to Know.

The documents revealed that Monsanto had known, years before the IARC classification, that glyphosate had cancer vulnerabilities. A 2014 internal email from Monsanto scientist William Heydens acknowledged the company's exposure: "while we have vulnerability in the area of epidemiology, we also have potential vulnerabilities in the other areas that IARC will consider, namely, exposure, genotox, and mode of action." Heydens was not describing a new discovery. He was describing what Monsanto had known for years and had chosen not to disclose or address.

In 1999, Heydens himself had declined to conduct tests that an outside expert had specifically advised were necessary to understand glyphosate's cancer risks. The tests were not done. The knowledge that the tests would have produced was not produced. What was not known could not be disclosed.

When the IARC classification was announced in 2015, Monsanto did not respond by investigating the concerns the IARC scientists had identified. It responded with what the Monsanto Papers document as an "unprecedented and harsh strategy" — in the words of Dr. Jonathan Samet, Dean of the Colorado School of Public Health, who described the company's approach in a 2019 peer-reviewed paper as paralleling "those used by the tobacco industry."

The strategy, documented in the internal emails, included:

Ghostwriting scientific literature. Monsanto arranged for scientific papers supporting glyphosate safety to be published under the names of ostensibly independent academic researchers. In one internal email, Heydens described the arrangement explicitly: the company could "ghost-write" certain reports, and outside scientists would "just edit and sign their names so to speak." He cited as an example a paper by Williams et al., published in 2000 in Regulatory Toxicology and Pharmacology, which had become a cornerstone reference for regulatory bodies, including the U.S. EPA, in their assessment of glyphosate safety. In November 2024, after the internal documents had made the ghostwriting relationship publicly undeniable, the journal retracted the Williams paper, citing "serious ethical concerns" including evidence that "Monsanto employees may have contributed to the writing of the article without acknowledgment."

Coordinating with EPA officials. The Monsanto Papers reveal a "particularly troubling relationship" with Jess Rowland, a senior EPA official who headed the agency's Cancer Assessment Review Committee and led the EPA's assessment of glyphosate's cancer risk. In a 2015 internal Monsanto email, Rowland is quoted saying he would try to block a planned Department of Health and Human Services review of glyphosate's safety: "If I can kill this I should get a medal." Monsanto's chief regulatory liaison, Dan Jenkins, wrote in the same period that Rowland "could be useful as we move forward with ongoing glyphosate defense." Rowland left the EPA shortly after the CARC report backing glyphosate's safety was made public.

Creating an Intelligence Fusion Center. The Monsanto Papers document the creation of what the company called an Intelligence Fusion Center — a monitoring operation that tracked journalists, activists, and scientists who were critical of the company. The tactics, according to researchers who analyzed the documents, mirrored those documented in the tobacco industry's campaigns against scientists studying smoking-related health risks.

The outcome of Monsanto's campaign was partial but significant. While the IARC's independent scientific classification of glyphosate as a probable carcinogen stands to this day, the EPA's determination — shaped by an agency official who was coordinating with Monsanto while running the assessment — concluded that glyphosate is "unlikely" to be carcinogenic. The EPA determination relied heavily on the Williams et al. paper, which has since been retracted for ghostwriting. As of 2025, the EPA's website still displays its "no risks of concern" determination for glyphosate — using language shaped by a review now withdrawn for ethical and scientific misconduct.

The litigation record tells a different story. By 2020, Bayer — which had acquired Monsanto in 2018 for $63 billion — had set aside more than $16 billion to cover glyphosate cancer litigation. By June 2020 it had agreed to pay more than $10 billion to settle approximately 100,000 claims. The total number of Roundup lawsuits filed against Monsanto/Bayer exceeded 192,000 by 2026. Three consecutive jury trials — Johnson v. Monsanto, Hardeman v.

Monsanto, and Pilliod v. Monsanto — produced verdicts finding that Roundup exposure was a substantial factor in causing plaintiffs' non-Hodgkin lymphoma, with juries in each case awarding significant punitive damages that were subsequently reduced by judges.

Bayer stopped selling Roundup to U.S. residential consumers in 2023. It continues selling glyphosate-based herbicides to commercial applicators and farmers. Glyphosate continues to be applied to the majority of corn, soy, and wheat crops in the United States. It is present in the food supply.

III. THE SEED MONOPOLY: PATENT LAW AND THE PRIVATIZATION OF LIFE

The chemical capture of the food supply required a biological foundation: the replacement of the open, diverse, farmer-controlled seed supply with a patented, corporate-owned seed system that made farmers dependent on purchasing new seed every year from a handful of companies.

This transformation was accomplished through the application of patent law to living organisms — a legal development that the U.S. Supreme Court enabled in 1980 in *Diamond v. Chakrabarty*, which held that genetically modified organisms could be patented. What followed was three decades of seed company consolidation and patent enforcement that restructured the foundation of American — and global — agriculture.

By the time the Supreme Court decided *Bowman v. Monsanto Co.* in 2013, the Public Patent Foundation had documented that Monsanto controlled 60% of the seed market for corn and soybeans, and that Roundup Ready herbicide-resistance technology had been planted in as much as 90% of all soybean crops in the United States. The Supreme Court's unanimous decision in *Bowman* confirmed the legal framework of that control: a farmer who buys patented seeds may not save and replant them without paying a fresh licensing fee for every season. The practice of seed saving — the foundational agricultural act that had sustained every human civilization for ten thousand years — became, in the context of patented seeds, patent infringement.

The mechanism of enforcement was documented in Monsanto's own legal filings and acknowledged in the company's public statements: Monsanto had filed suit against 145 individual U.S. farmers for patent infringement and related claims, proceeding through trial against eleven of them. The company employed investigators to monitor fields and collect samples. The legal costs of defending against Monsanto's patent enforcement actions were sufficient to deter even farmers who believed they had a legitimate defense.

The broader consequences were documented by organizations including the Center for Food Safety and Save Our Seeds: the seed monopoly had reduced the diversity of available seed varieties, raised seed prices, limited scientific research on alternative varieties, and made the industrial agricultural system — dependent on annual seed purchases, on the herbicide systems the patented seeds were designed to require, and on the chemical inputs those systems necessitated — structurally resistant to disruption or independent development.

The farmers who planted Monsanto's Roundup Ready seeds bought those seeds under license. They then purchased Roundup — Monsanto's proprietary glyphosate herbicide — to manage weeds in fields where crops resistant to glyphosate had been planted. The seed and the chemical were a system, each requiring the other, and both owned by the same company. By the time Bayer acquired Monsanto for $63 billion in 2018, the integration of seed patents and chemical dependencies had created an agricultural infrastructure whose basic inputs — the seed to plant and the chemical to protect it — were controlled at the corporate level.

Justice Clarence Thomas, who wrote no opinion in *Bowman v. Monsanto*, had previously served as a corporate attorney for Monsanto before his appointment to the Supreme Court. He did not recuse himself from the case.

IV. THE PROCESSED FOOD SYSTEM: ENGINEERING ADDICTION AND MANUFACTURING CHRONIC ILLNESS

The dietary guidelines that the sugar industry's purchased science had shaped recommended reducing fat and increasing carbohydrates. The food industry responded — not by producing foods that were genuinely more nutritious, but by producing foods that met the letter of the low-fat recommendation while systematically replacing natural fats with refined carbohydrates, added sugars, industrial seed oils, and synthetic additives engineered to make food as palatable — and as compulsively consumed — as possible.

The science of what the food industry calls "hyperpalatability" is documented in industry research and in the investigative work of journalists and researchers who have obtained internal documents. The goal was identified explicitly in industry communications: to engineer foods that override the human body's natural satiety mechanisms, producing consumption patterns that bear no relationship to nutritional need.

The specific mechanisms — the precise combinations of salt, sugar, and fat that produce the highest "bliss point," the texture engineering that triggers rapid consumption, the caloric density calibrated to produce reward without satiation — are documented in the research of food scientists like Howard Moskowitz, whose work for Campbell Soup, Coca-Cola, and other major food manufacturers on optimizing consumer response is described in Moskowitz's own published presentations and in Michael Moss's *Salt Sugar Fat* (Random House, 2013), which drew on internal industry documents and extensive interviews with food scientists who had conducted this research.

The consequences are in the public health data. From 1980 — the year the first federal Dietary Guidelines were published — to 1997, total daily calorie consumption per capita increased by more than 500 calories, primarily driven by increased carbohydrate intake. From 1980 to 2020, the prevalence of obesity in American adults increased from approximately 15% to 42%. Type 2 diabetes, which had affected approximately 1% of the American population in 1960, affected approximately 11% by 2020. Metabolic syndrome — a cluster of conditions including elevated blood sugar, high blood pressure, excess abdominal fat, and abnormal cholesterol levels — is estimated to affect approximately one-third of American adults.

These are not the outcomes of a well-intentioned dietary advice system that happened to produce unintended consequences. They are the outcomes documented in the Sugar Research Foundation's own papers from 1954: the recognition that a low-fat dietary regime would increase per-capita sugar consumption by more than one-third. The recognition that the low-fat recommendation, if adopted, would serve the sugar industry's financial interests. The decision to fund the research that would produce that recommendation.

The food system that the dietary guidelines built, the seed patents enforced, and the chemical agriculture deployed — managed by a USDA whose dietary guidelines process is subject to the same industry capture documented at the FDA in Chapter 7 — is a system that produces chronic illness at the population level. Chronic illness requires medical management. Medical management is pharmaceutical product delivery. The food system and the pharmaceutical system are not separate industries that happen to share a customer base. They are sequential stages of the same apparatus.

V. THE USDA CAPTURE: HOW THE AGENCY THAT MANAGES THE FOOD SUPPLY WAS MANAGED BY THE FOOD INDUSTRY

The USDA is simultaneously the agency responsible for promoting American agricultural production and the agency responsible for setting federal dietary guidelines — a structural conflict of interest whose consequences are visible in every edition of the *Dietary Guidelines for Americans* published since 1980.

The Dietary Guidelines Advisory Committee — the body of scientific experts that reviews the evidence and makes recommendations to the USDA and HHS before each edition — operates under a process that allows the food industry to submit public comments, attend hearings, and lobby committee members during the comment period. In the 2020-2025 guidelines process, a letter from The Nutrition Coalition to the USDA and HHS documented that whistleblowers on the Dietary Guidelines Advisory Committee had reported inadequate time to complete scientific reviews, deletion of some reviews and addition of others without required public notice, exclusion of important scientific evidence including studies of low-carbohydrate diets, and rejection of reforms recommended by the National Academy of Sciences.

The food industry's influence on federal dietary policy is also exercised through direct financial relationships with the regulatory process. The food and beverage industry has contributed close to $200 million to Political Action Committees and congressional members over recent years, according to documented campaign finance records. These contributions flow disproportionately to members of the congressional committees that oversee the USDA and the dietary guidelines process.

The result is a dietary guidance system that has consistently protected the financial interests of the industries it nominally regulates. The 1985 edition of the Dietary Guidelines dropped even the conditional language about sugar and diabetes, declaring unambiguously that "too much sugar in your diet does not cause diabetes" — despite the fact that USDA researchers at the Carbohydrate Nutrition Laboratory were, at the same time, producing research that contradicted this conclusion. In the 2020-2025 edition, the government rejected its own scientific advisory committee's recommendation for lower sugar targets.

The same industry that funded Project 226 in 1965 was still shaping federal dietary advice in 2020. The investment compounded across six decades.

VI. THE COMPLETE PICTURE

The food system documented in this chapter — the purchased dietary science, the chemical agriculture built on suppressed safety data, the seed patents that ended the farmer's relationship with the seed, the processed food engineered for addiction rather than nourishment, the federal agency structurally incapable of protecting the public from the industries it promotes — is not a system that failed to provide the nourishment it promised.

It is a system that succeeded at what it was actually built to do.

The sugar industry recognized in 1954 that a low-fat dietary recommendation would increase sugar consumption by more than one-third. It then spent $50,000 in 1965 to purchase the Harvard review that would produce that recommendation. The investment worked.

Monsanto knew internally that glyphosate had cancer vulnerabilities. It declined to conduct the tests that would have quantified those vulnerabilities. It ghostwrote the literature that regulatory agencies used to clear the chemical. It coordinated with an EPA official who offered to "kill" a government safety review. The investment worked — for decades, until the litigation forced the documents into the open.

The seed patents eliminated the farmer's biological independence and created structural dependency on an integrated chemical-seed system. The Roundup Ready soybean required Roundup. The Roundup required Roundup Ready seeds. Both belonged to the same company.

And the processed food engineered at the "bliss point" — formulated specifically to override satiety, to produce consumption beyond nutritional need, to create behavioral patterns that resemble addiction — produced the chronic illness whose pharmaceutical management is documented in Chapter 7.

Chapter 7 showed that the FDA became dependent on the pharmaceutical industry it was supposed to regulate. This chapter shows what that pharmaceutical dependency was built on: a food system engineered to produce the chronic illness that pharmaceutical management exists to address.

The pen has many rooms. This chapter documents the one that feeds it.

"You shall have them for food."

That was the provision. What was done to it is what this chapter documents.

PRIMARY SOURCES FOR THIS CHAPTER

Sugar Industry — Internal Documents and Peer-Reviewed Analysis:

- Kearns, C.E., Schmidt, L.A., and Glantz, S.A. "Sugar Industry and Coronary Heart Disease Research: A Historical Analysis of Internal Industry Documents." *JAMA Internal Medicine*, November 1, 2016; 176(11):1680-1685. doi: 10.1001/jamainternmed.2016.5394. The landmark peer-reviewed paper documenting the Sugar Research Foundation's funding and direction of the Harvard review. Available at PMC (pmc.ncbi.nlm.nih.gov, PMC5099084) and at jamanetwork.com.

- UCSF SugarScience press release, September 12, 2016. Available at sugarscience.ucsf.edu. Provides additional context and quotes from the study's authors.

- Original industry documents analyzed in the paper, found in public archives: correspondence between the Sugar Research Foundation and Harvard researchers at the Francis A. Countway Library of Medicine and the University of Illinois Archives.

USDA Dietary Guidelines — Primary Documents and Capture Evidence:

- *Dietary Goals for the United States*, U.S. Senate Select Committee on Nutrition and Human Needs, January 1977. The McGovern Report. Available through the National Agricultural Library.

- *Dietary Guidelines for Americans*, 1980-2020 editions. All editions available at dietaryguidelines.gov.

- Whistleblower letter to USDA and HHS from The Nutrition Coalition, June 2020. Documents reported misconduct in the Dietary Guidelines Advisory Committee process.

- Wikipedia documentation of the 2020-2025 guidelines cycle confirming the federal government's rejection of its advisory committee's recommendation on sugar consumption targets.

Monsanto Papers — Litigation Discovery Documents:

- U.S. District Court for the Northern District of California, *In Re: Roundup Products Liability Litigation* (MDL). The foundational litigation producing the Monsanto Papers. Key cases: *Johnson v. Monsanto* (2018), *Hardeman v. Monsanto* (2019), *Pilliod v. Monsanto* (2019).

- Monsanto Papers archive maintained by Wisner Baum law firm at wisnerbaum.com/monsanto-papers and by U.S. Right to Know at usrtk.org/monsanto-papers. Contains the court-ordered released internal emails, including the Heydens "ghost-write" email and the Rowland "I should get a medal" email.

- "Suborning science for profit: Monsanto, glyphosate, and private science research misconduct." *Research Policy*, 2021. Peer-reviewed analysis of the Monsanto Papers ghostwriting practices. Available at sciencedirect.com.

- "Internal documents reveal pesticide industry science denial and manipulation: glyphosate case study." U.S. Right to Know, drawing on the litigation documents. Available at usrtk.org.

- Samet, J. (2019). Academic paper documenting Monsanto's post-IARC strategy as paralleling tobacco industry tactics.

Williams et al. Retraction:

- Retraction notice, *Regulatory Toxicology and Pharmacology*, November 28, 2024. Co-editor-in-chief Martin van den Berg documenting the retraction of Williams et al. (2000) for "serious ethical concerns" including undisclosed Monsanto authorship. Reported by *Science* magazine (AAAS), December 5, 2024.

IARC Classification:

- International Agency for Research on Cancer (IARC), Monograph 112: Glyphosate. 2015. The WHO agency's classification of glyphosate as a Group 2A probable human carcinogen. Available at iarc.fr.

Seed Monopoly — Court Records:

- *Bowman v. Monsanto Co.*, 569 U.S. 278 (2013). The Supreme Court's unanimous decision. Full text at supremecourt.gov and at supreme.justia.com.

- *Monsanto legal cases*, documented at en.wikipedia.org/wiki/Monsanto_legal_cases. Summarizes the 145 farmer lawsuits filed by Monsanto for patent infringement.

- Public Patent Foundation documentation that Monsanto controlled 60% of the corn and soybean seed market and that Roundup Ready technology had been planted in approximately 90% of U.S. soybean crops. Cited in *Bowman* litigation filings.

Bayer Settlement:

- Bayer AG public statements and investor communications, 2020-2021. Documenting the $16 billion litigation reserve and $10+ billion settlement commitment for glyphosate cancer claims.

The reader is encouraged to begin with the Kearns, Schmidt, and Glantz paper in JAMA Internal Medicine — it is available free of charge through the NIH's PubMed Central — and with the Monsanto Papers archive at usrtk.org. Both are primary documents that require no intermediary. Read the emails. Read the study. The evidence does not require interpretation.

Chapter 9: The Childhood Vaccine Schedule

Liability, Mandates, and the Questions That Were Never Asked

"Let the children come to me; do not hinder them, for to such belongs the kingdom of God."

— Mark 10:14

This chapter will be read by people on every point of the spectrum of opinion about childhood vaccines. Some will arrive believing the current schedule is among the greatest achievements of modern medicine. Some will arrive believing it is among the greatest harms ever systematically inflicted on children. Most will arrive somewhere between these positions, carrying a mixture of trust and unease they cannot fully articulate.

This chapter will not tell any of them what to believe. It will tell all of them what the documented record shows — what Congress did in 1986, what the law required afterward, what the government admitted it never did, what the schedule looked like in 1983 and what it looks like today, what the compensation program has paid and to whom, and what questions about the safety of individual vaccines and the combined schedule remain unanswered not because the science is settled but because the studies were never conducted.

The reader who finishes this chapter will be better equipped to evaluate the evidence than they were before they began. That is the chapter's only ambition.

I. 1986: THE YEAR LIABILITY ENDED

To understand the childhood vaccine schedule as it exists today, you must begin with a single piece of legislation and a single date.

November 14, 1986. President Ronald Reagan signs the National Childhood Vaccine Injury Act — Public Law 99-660 — into law as part of a broader health bill.

The context for the law is documented in its own legislative record. In the late 1970s and early 1980s, a wave of lawsuits against vaccine manufacturers — primarily related to the pertussis component of the DPT vaccine and its alleged link to brain injury — had created a crisis in the vaccine market. Liability insurance for vaccine manufacturers became difficult to obtain. Multiple manufacturers stopped producing vaccines. By 1985, only one company was still manufacturing pertussis vaccine in the United States. That company was considering withdrawal from the market as well.

Congress faced a genuine dilemma: the liability system that was supposed to protect children injured by vaccines was simultaneously threatening to eliminate the vaccines themselves. The National Childhood Vaccine Injury Act was Congress's solution.

The solution had two parts, documented in the law's text.

The first part eliminated the manufacturer's direct civil liability for vaccine injuries. Under the Act, a person injured by a covered vaccine could no longer file a civil lawsuit against the manufacturer in state or federal court without first exhausting the federal compensation program. The Supreme Court's 2011 ruling in *Bruesewitz v. Wyeth* extended this protection further, holding that even claims of defective vaccine design — the category that most vaccine injury lawsuits had used — were barred by the Act. Vaccine manufacturers are shielded from liability so long as they comply with regulatory requirements and do not commit fraud, criminal acts, or intentionally withhold information from patients.

The second part created the National Vaccine Injury Compensation Program — a no-fault alternative system funded not by manufacturers but by a $0.75 excise tax on every dose of covered vaccine purchased. Claims would be adjudicated by the U.S. Court of Federal Claims, with special masters hearing petitions and awarding compensation from the trust fund.

The law's logic was explicit: since vaccine manufacturers were being relieved of the financial incentive to ensure the safety of their products — the fear of losing in court — the federal government would assume the responsibility of ensuring vaccine safety in their place. Congress embedded this responsibility directly in the statute. Section 2127 of the Act required the Secretary of Health and Human Services to submit a biannual report to Congress detailing improvements made in the preceding two years to vaccine safety. The report was to begin in 1988 and continue every two years thereafter.

The vaccine manufacturers received their protection. What the children received, in the law's own terms, was the government's promise to take safety seriously in the manufacturers' place.

That promise will be addressed in Section IV of this chapter.

II. THE SCHEDULE: WHAT CHANGED AND WHEN

In 1983 — three years before the liability shield was enacted — the recommended childhood immunization schedule for American children consisted of 11 doses of 4 vaccines, protecting against 7 diseases: diphtheria, tetanus, pertussis, measles, mumps, rubella, and polio. This was the schedule that had been in place, with minor modifications, for the preceding generation.

The schedule that exists in 2024 — four decades later — recommends 88 doses of 16 vaccines from birth through 18 years of age.

The expansion did not happen immediately after 1986. The historical record of vaccine additions to the schedule documents the trajectory:

By 1989, Haemophilus influenzae type b (Hib) vaccine had been added, bringing the schedule to 12 doses of 5 vaccines. By 1995, hepatitis B — recommended beginning on the day of birth — and varicella (chickenpox) had been added, expanding the schedule to 19 doses of 6 vaccines. The following decade added hepatitis A, pneumococcal conjugate, rotavirus, meningococcal, HPV, and an expanded influenza recommendation for all ages. By 2023, the COVID-19 vaccine had been added to the schedule.

Each addition to the schedule follows the same pathway: a vaccine manufacturer completes clinical trials and submits to the FDA for approval, the FDA reviews the application and approves the vaccine, the Advisory Committee on Immunization Practices reviews the evidence and makes a recommendation for routine use, the CDC director adopts the recommendation, and the recommendation becomes the standard of care against which pediatricians and health plans operate.

This pathway has produced demonstrable public health benefits. Diseases that once killed and disabled thousands of American children annually — polio, measles at epidemic scale, Haemophilus meningitis — have been dramatically reduced or virtually eliminated in the United States. This is not in dispute and this chapter does not dispute it.

What this chapter examines is the institutional architecture that governs the pathway — the liability structure, the advisory committee process, the safety testing methodology, and the oversight requirements — and what the documented record reveals about whether that architecture has functioned as Congress intended.

III. VICP: THE COMPENSATION RECORD

Since the National Vaccine Injury Compensation Program began accepting petitions in 1988, the federal government has paid more than $5.2 billion in compensation to approximately 10,000 individuals and families for vaccine-related injuries and deaths. The funding for these payments has come entirely from the $0.75 per dose excise tax — not from the manufacturers whose products caused the injuries.

This is a documented fact, available at HRSA's public data portal at hrsa.gov/vaccine-compensation/data.

The VICP is a no-fault system, which means compensation is available without proving that the manufacturer did anything wrong. The Vaccine Injury Table maintained by HHS lists specific vaccines, associated adverse events, and the timeframes in which those events must occur to qualify for presumptive compensation. If an injury matches a table entry within the specified timeframe, the government presumes causation and awards compensation without requiring the petitioner to prove it.

Several things about the compensation record deserve noting.

First, COVID-19 vaccines are not covered by the VICP. Under the PREP Act — the Public Readiness and Emergency Preparedness Act — COVID-19 vaccines were covered instead by the Countermeasures Injury Compensation Program (CICP), which has significantly more restricted compensation criteria, lower maximum awards, no attorney fee coverage for unsuccessful claims, and a higher burden of proof. The population that received the most recently deployed novel vaccine technology did so under a compensation framework substantially less protective than the one that covers the vaccines that preceded it.

Second, the $5.2 billion total represents only the claims that were filed and compensated. The VICP's own data and academic analysis suggest that the rate of adverse event reporting and compensation claiming is a fraction of actual adverse events. VAERS — the Vaccine Adverse Event Reporting System — is a passive surveillance system; healthcare providers report adverse events voluntarily, and the CDC explicitly states that VAERS data cannot establish causation. The number of people who experience a vaccine-related adverse event and either do not report it, do not connect it to a vaccine, or do not navigate the compensation process is unknown and has not been rigorously studied.

Third, the compensation record documents that vaccine injuries are real, that they occur, and that the government has accepted legal responsibility for paying for them. This is not a contested point. The question the compensation record raises — and that the following sections address — is whether the institutional mechanisms designed to minimize those injuries have functioned as intended.

IV. THE SAFETY PROMISE THAT WAS NEVER KEPT

Return to Section 2127 of the 1986 Act: the requirement that HHS submit biannual reports to Congress on improvements to vaccine safety.

The first report was due in 1988. A new report was due every two years thereafter — 1990, 1992, 1994, 1996, 1998, through to the present.

In August 2017, the Informed Consent Action Network — ICAN — filed a Freedom of Information Act request with HHS seeking copies of these biannual reports. For eight months, HHS provided no substantive response. ICAN filed a lawsuit in the U.S. District Court for the Southern District of New York, demanding either the production of the reports or an admission that they did not exist.

HHS conceded. The biannual vaccine safety reports to Congress — required by federal law since 1988, the explicit legislative quid pro quo for the liability shield granted to manufacturers — had never been produced. Not a single one. The Court entered an order confirming HHS's concession.

ICAN announced the outcome in a press release dated September 14, 2018, available through PRNewswire's public archive.

The Task Force on Safer Childhood Vaccines — the body the 1986 Act had created to do the actual work of improving vaccine safety — was disbanded by HHS in 1998, ten years after it was created and twelve years before the schedule would double in size.

HHS's public posture throughout this period was one of vigorous commitment to vaccine safety. It spent billions annually promoting vaccine uptake. It generated a steady stream of reports on how to increase vaccination rates. It defended against vaccine injury claims in the compensation program. What it did not do, as the court record now confirms, was fulfill the specific statutory obligation Congress had placed on it as the condition of granting manufacturers their liability shield.

The 1986 Act's logic was: manufacturers give up their liability incentive to ensure safety; HHS assumes that responsibility instead. What the court record documents is that HHS accepted the arrangement's benefits for manufacturers while failing to fulfill its own end of the exchange.

The Task Force on Safer Childhood Vaccines was reinstated by HHS in August 2025, following a lawsuit filed by Children's Health Defense. It had been disbanded for twenty-seven years.

V. THE ADVISORY COMMITTEE AND CONFLICTS OF INTEREST: WHAT THE RECORD SHOWS

The Advisory Committee on Immunization Practices — ACIP — is the body that recommends vaccines for addition to the childhood schedule. Its recommendations, when adopted by the CDC director, become the effective standard of care for American pediatric medicine, determine which vaccines are covered by major insurance programs, and inform the vaccine requirements that states attach to school enrollment.

The documented history of ACIP conflicts of interest is a matter of congressional record, not allegation.

In June 2000, the Committee on Government Reform of the U.S. House of Representatives held a hearing titled "FACA: Conflicts of Interest and Vaccine Development — Preserving the Integrity of the Process." The hearing record, available in full at govinfo.gov (CHRG-106hhrg73042), documents the following specific cases:

Dr. John Modlin was the chairman of ACIP's rotavirus working group and voted on eight matters pertaining to the rotavirus vaccine recommendation, including recommending it for routine use and inclusion in the Vaccines for Children program. Dr. Modlin owned $26,000 in Merck stock — one of the largest vaccine manufacturers — and served on Merck's immunization advisory board. He did not divest his stock until the year of the congressional hearing.

Dr. Paul Offit held a patent on a rotavirus vaccine and received grant funding from Merck to develop it. He also disclosed that he was paid by the pharmaceutical industry to travel and teach doctors that vaccines are safe. Dr. Offit voted on three rotavirus issues, including recommending the rotavirus vaccine for the Vaccines for Children program.

At least 6 of the 10 individuals who participated in the working group for the rotavirus vaccine — the closed-door subgroup that did the detailed deliberative work before full committee votes — had financial ties to pharmaceutical companies developing rotavirus vaccines.

The congressional record also notes a structural problem that the conflicts of interest at the full-committee level understated: members who were prohibited from voting in the full committee due to conflicts of interest were nonetheless permitted to participate in working groups that met outside public scrutiny, where the detailed development of recommendations occurred.

The JAMA 2025 study referenced in the current ACIP Wikipedia entry documents that conflicts of interest among ACIP members declined significantly after 2000 — from a peak of 42.8% in 2000 to approximately 5% by 2024 — primarily due to heightened public scrutiny following the congressional hearing and subsequent reform efforts. The decline is real and documented. It is also true that the schedule expanded from approximately 30 doses in 2000 to 88 doses in 2023, and that the pattern of conflicts documented in the congressional record preceded and likely influenced recommendations made during the period of greatest schedule expansion.

The current CDC disclosure database — launched in March 2025 at cdc.gov/acip/disclosures/by-member.html — makes historical ACIP conflict disclosures publicly searchable for the period from 2000 to 2024. The reader can examine the record directly.

VI. THE TRIAL METHODOLOGY QUESTION

Before a vaccine can be added to the childhood schedule it must receive FDA approval. FDA approval requires clinical trial data demonstrating that the vaccine is safe and effective. The nature of the control group used in those trials — what the trial participants who did not receive the vaccine actually received — is a question the documented record shows is more complex than is often acknowledged.

This complexity is genuinely contested scientific territory, and this chapter will describe it accurately rather than advocate for a position.

The mainstream scientific position, articulated by the American Academy of Pediatrics, the CDC, and researchers who have compiled systematic reviews of vaccine clinical trial data, is that childhood vaccines have been extensively tested in randomized controlled trials, many of which used inert saline placebos, and that the accumulated safety evidence across pre-licensure and post-licensure surveillance is robust. A 2025 systematic review of vaccine randomized controlled trial literature identified more than 274 such trials, of which approximately 133 used inert placebo controls.

The critical question raised by researchers and advocates who have examined the trial record in detail concerns a different category of vaccines — those for which the control group received not an inert saline placebo but either an aluminum adjuvant preparation (the same adjuvant as in the vaccine, without the antigen), another licensed vaccine, or a combination. The Gardasil (HPV) clinical trial data, documented in FDA approval records, provides the clearest example: in the primary trials, 15,706 individuals received the quadrivalent Gardasil vaccine. A control group of 594 individuals received a true saline placebo. A second control group of 13,023 individuals received the aluminum adjuvant component of the vaccine — the same adjuvant critics have identified as a potential source of adverse reactions — without the viral antigen. Critics argue that using an active adjuvant as the primary control obscures the actual adverse event rate because both groups are experiencing the adjuvant's effects, making the vaccine appear safer than a true saline comparison would reveal.

The mainstream response to this argument is that using the adjuvant as a control allows researchers to isolate the immunological effect of the antigen specifically, which is the scientifically relevant comparison — and that the combined pre-licensure and post-licensure safety record provides adequate evidence of safety.

What this chapter documents — with precision, because precision matters here — is the following:

The pre-licensure safety trials for individual vaccines were not designed to study the combined effects of administering multiple vaccines simultaneously, which is the actual clinical situation children face when they receive several vaccines at a single well-child visit. No pre-licensure trial has studied whether the combination of all vaccines recommended in the first year of life produces different safety outcomes than any individual vaccine produces in isolation. This is not a disputed fact. The studies were not conducted because pre-licensure trials are designed to evaluate individual products, not combinations.

The post-licensure surveillance systems — VAERS, the Vaccine Safety Datalink, the Clinical Immunization Safety Assessment Project — exist in part to detect safety signals that pre-licensure trials are too small or too short to identify. VAERS is explicitly described by the CDC as a hypothesis-generating system that cannot establish causation. The Vaccine Safety Datalink is a more rigorous observational database but covers only a subset of the population.

The documented record — from the court confirmation that HHS never filed its required biannual safety reports, to the congressional testimony about ACIP conflicts of interest in the period of greatest schedule expansion, to the absence of combined-schedule safety studies — establishes that the institutional mechanisms designed to ensure the childhood schedule is as safe as possible did not operate as Congress intended during the decades when the schedule tripled in size.

What the evidence does not establish — and this chapter will not assert — is that specific vaccines in the schedule cause specific harms at specific rates in the general population. The honest evidentiary position is more precise than that: the questions were not asked with the rigor the scale of the program warranted. That is not the same as saying the answers would be alarming. It is saying that the answers were not sought.

VII. WHAT WAS STUDIED AND WHAT WASN'T

The 1954 Francis Field Trial — the polio vaccine trial — enrolled more than 400,000 American children, half of whom received an inert placebo. It remains one of the largest randomized controlled trials in medical history. The urgency of polio as a public health catastrophe justified the scale of investigation before the vaccine was deployed to the entire child population.

The childhood vaccine schedule that has been assembled in the decades since does not have an equivalent study. No trial has enrolled hundreds of thousands of children to compare the combined health outcomes — not merely the incidence of targeted infectious diseases but all-cause morbidity, chronic illness rates, and long-term developmental outcomes — of children who received the full recommended schedule against children who received none of it or an alternative schedule.

The absence of this study is not a scientific scandal in itself. Conducting such a trial would be extremely difficult, would take decades, and would raise genuine ethical concerns about withholding vaccines with demonstrated protection from infectious disease. These are real constraints, honestly acknowledged.

What is documented in the record is that the question of whether the expansion of the schedule from 11 doses in 1983 to 88 doses in 2024 has affected rates of childhood chronic illness — which have risen substantially during the same period — has not been answered by a study designed to answer it. The correlation between schedule expansion and rising rates of childhood allergies, asthma, autoimmune conditions, and neurodevelopmental disorders is real and documented in public health data. Whether the correlation reflects causation, and to what degree, is genuinely unknown because the studies that would answer the question have not been conducted.

The correlation does not prove causation. The absence of the study does not prove harm. But the documented institutional failures described in this chapter — the disbanded safety task force, the unfiled safety reports, the conflicted advisory committee, the absence of combined-schedule safety research — are the context in which the rising rates of childhood chronic illness must be evaluated. The rising rates cannot be evaluated in a vacuum any more than the opioid crisis can be evaluated without understanding the FDA's capture documented in Chapter 7.

VIII. COVID-19 AND THE SCHEDULE

In 2023, the COVID-19 vaccine was added to the recommended childhood immunization schedule by ACIP and the CDC director.

The addition occurred after the vaccines had received Emergency Use Authorization — not full FDA licensure — for children down to 6 months of age. The clinical trial data supporting authorization in young children involved smaller populations observed over shorter periods than the trials that had historically preceded schedule inclusion. The long-term safety data that would normally accumulate over years before schedule inclusion was not available because the vaccines had not existed for years.

COVID-19 vaccines are not covered by the National Vaccine Injury Compensation Program. Individuals injured by a COVID-19 vaccine — including children for whom the vaccine is now on the recommended schedule — must seek compensation through the CICP, which since 2020 had approved fewer than 15% of claims filed and whose maximum compensation is lower than VICP's.

The addition of COVID-19 vaccines to the childhood schedule illustrates in compressed form the structural problem this chapter documents: a vaccine developed and authorized on an emergency timeline, with limited long-term safety data, added to a schedule that children need to comply with for school enrollment in many states, covered by a compensation program with significantly more restricted terms than the one covering every other vaccine on the schedule.

The children who receive the COVID-19 vaccine as part of the routine childhood schedule receive it under materially different institutional protections than the children who received the hepatitis B vaccine in 1991, the varicella vaccine in 1995, or the HPV vaccine in 2006.

IX. THE LEGITIMATE QUESTION

This chapter has documented the following from the primary source record:

The 1986 Act removed manufacturer liability and placed the responsibility for vaccine safety on HHS. HHS accepted that responsibility and then failed to fulfill its specific statutory obligations — never filing the biannual safety reports, disbanding the safety task force in 1998 — for decades. The schedule tripled in size during the period when the safety task force was disbanded and the safety reports were not filed. The advisory committee that recommended the additions to the schedule had documented conflicts of interest, peaking at 42.8% of members in 2000, during the period of greatest expansion. The pre-licensure trials for individual vaccines were not designed to study combined-schedule effects. No large-scale study has examined long-term health outcomes across vaccinated and unvaccinated populations. Children injured by COVID-19 vaccines, now on the recommended schedule, have access to significantly more restricted compensation than children injured by other schedule vaccines.

None of this documentation constitutes proof that specific vaccines are harmful to specific children at specific rates. The evidentiary standard for that conclusion requires studies that have not been conducted.

What the documentation does constitute is a precise indictment of the institutional architecture that was supposed to ensure the safety of the program. The manufacturers were protected. The safety obligation was accepted. The safety obligation was not fulfilled. The schedule expanded. The questions that should have been asked were not asked.

The children who received the vaccines during this period were not consulted about the adequacy of the institutional oversight under which their schedule was built. Neither were their parents, most of whom trusted the schedule because they trusted the institutions behind it. That trust was extended in good faith. Whether it was warranted in every specific instance is the question the missing studies — the ones the disbanded task force should have been generating — would have answered.

Let the children come to me; do not hinder them.

The one who spoke those words did not say: let the children come to me only after the institutional conflicts of interest are resolved and the biannual safety reports have been filed. He did not condition his welcome on the completion of the combined-schedule safety study. The children belong to him regardless of what the institutional record shows about the adults who were charged with their protection.

That is not a political statement. It is a reminder of where the weight of this evidence ultimately falls — not on an abstraction called public health policy, but on specific children, in specific families, who deserved better from every institution this chapter documents.

PRIMARY SOURCES FOR THIS CHAPTER

Legislation and Court Records:

- National Childhood Vaccine Injury Act of 1986, Public Law 99-660. Full text at congress.gov (H.R.5546, 99th Congress) and through the National Academies at nationalacademies.org (Appendix C of *Priorities for the National Vaccine Plan*). Section 2127 contains the biannual reporting requirement. Section 2122 contains the liability shield provisions.

- *Bruesewitz v. Wyeth*, 562 U.S. 223 (2011). The Supreme Court decision extending the liability shield to design defect claims. Full text at supremecourt.gov.

- ICAN v. HHS, U.S. District Court for the Southern District of New York (2018). The court order confirming HHS's concession that no biannual vaccine safety reports exist. The outcome was announced in a press release dated September 14, 2018, available at PRNewswire (search "ICAN HHS vaccine safety 2018").

- *Bowman v. Monsanto Co.* citation noted for parallel structure in

Chapter 8; the ICAN case is the Chapter 9 equivalent.

VICP Compensation Data:

- HRSA Vaccine Injury Compensation Data. Available at hrsa.gov/vaccine-compensation/data. The official federal record of claims filed, compensated, and amounts paid since 1988.

- HRSA About the National Vaccine Injury Compensation Program. Available at hrsa.gov/vaccine-compensation/about. Documents the $0.75/dose excise tax funding mechanism.

- HRSA FAQ on VICP and COVID-19 vaccines. Available at hrsa.gov/vaccine-compensation/faq. Confirms COVID-19 vaccines are covered by CICP, not VICP.

Congressional Record:

- "FACA: Conflicts of Interest and Vaccine Development — Preserving the Integrity of the Process." Committee on Government Reform, U.S. House of Representatives, Hearing, 2000. Full text at govinfo.gov, document identifier CHRG-106hhrg73042. Documents the Modlin, Offit, and working group conflict cases in congressional testimony.

- ACIP Conflicts of Interest Disclosure Database. Available at cdc.gov/acip/disclosures/by-member.html. All ACIP member conflict disclosures from 2000 to 2024 are publicly searchable.

Schedule History:

- CDC Recommended Childhood Immunization Schedules, historical archives. Available at cdc.gov/vaccines/schedules and through CDC's historical schedule documentation.

- Documented comparison: 11 doses of 4 vaccines in 1983 (AAP 1983 schedule) versus 88 doses of 16 vaccines in the current schedule. Historical schedule documentation available at vaxopedia.org/2019/07/09/vaccine-schedules-from-the-1940s-to-2019 with AAP source citations.

Clinical Trial Methodology:

- FDA clinical trial data for Gardasil (HPV quadrivalent vaccine, Merck), documenting the trial group distribution: 15,706 receiving vaccine, 13,023 receiving aluminum adjuvant control, 594 receiving inert saline placebo. Available through FDA's biologics approval documents for Gardasil (BLA 125126).

- Martínez-Lavin, M. and Amezcua-Guerra, L. Peer-reviewed analysis of HPV vaccine clinical trials, published July 2017. Documents the distribution of control group types across 16 HPV vaccine randomized trials.

- CIDRAP systematic review of vaccine randomized controlled trial literature, 2025. Documents 274 vaccine RCTs of which 133 used inert placebo controls.

Task Force Reinstatement:

- Children's Health Defense press release and reporting, August 2025. Documents HHS's reinstatement of the Task Force on Safer Childhood Vaccines, disbanded since 1998, following a CHD lawsuit. Available at childrenshealthdefense.org.

- ICAN letter to HHS Secretary Kennedy, FDA Commissioner Makary, and NIH Director Bhattacharya, March 2026. Documenting the task force's statutory obligations. Available at icandecide.org.

Conflicts of Interest — Peer-Reviewed Documentation:

- JAMA study on ACIP conflicts of interest, August 2025. Published in JAMA (specific citation: University of Southern California Schaeffer Center research, published August 2025). Confirms peak conflicts of 42.8% in 2000, decline to 5% by 2024. Coverage available at schaeffer.usc.edu.

The primary sources for this chapter are available in the public record. The congressional hearing transcript at govinfo.gov is particularly important — it is verbatim testimony from members of Congress and the experts they called, in an official federal record. The ICAN press release documents a court outcome. The HRSA data is the federal government's own compensation record. None of these sources require trust in an advocacy position. They are official documents. Read them.

Chapter 10: The Epstein Network

Enforcement, Compromise, and Institutional Protection at Scale

"It would be better for him if a millstone were hung around his neck and he were cast into the sea than that he should cause one of these little ones to stumble."

— Luke 17:2

The verse above is not a metaphor. It is the judgment of Jesus Christ on a specific category of crime. He did not say it is unfortunate, or that it should be punished, or that society should look into it. He said the man who does this would be better off drowned. The chapter that follows documents what was done, to whom, by whom, and through what institutional protections it was sustained for decades.

The documentation is what it is. The judgment was already rendered.

I. WHAT THE NETWORK WAS

Jeffrey Epstein was not primarily a sex trafficker who happened to know powerful people. That framing — the one that dominated early coverage and allowed the story to be contained as a scandal of individual moral failure — is precisely backward.

What the primary source record establishes, across the trial record of *United States v. Maxwell*, the Department of Justice's own Office of Professional Responsibility report on the non-prosecution agreement, the Miami Herald's court-document-based investigative series, and the internal emails produced by institutions that accepted Epstein's funding, is this:

Epstein operated a sophisticated intelligence-connected network whose documented function included the systematic compromise and management of elite compliance across medicine, science, finance, politics, media, and academia. The trafficking of minors was simultaneously the network's most vicious crime and its most effective operational instrument — because the individuals who participated in it, or who knew of it and said nothing, were thereafter subject to the network's control in ways that shaped their institutional behavior for years.

The people who built the apparatus documented in this book — the regulatory capture, the food system, the childhood health infrastructure, the global coordination — operated within a world where this network functioned as an enforcement and containment mechanism. The people most capable of disrupting the apparatus were the people most comprehensively inside the network's reach. That is not a coincidence. It is the network's design.

What the documented record shows, and what this chapter presents from the primary sources, is an operation that sustained itself for decades across multiple federal jurisdictions, survived at least one documented federal investigation that produced an extraordinary non-prosecution agreement, embedded itself in the most prestigious scientific and academic institutions in the world, and ended not because any institution disrupted it but because journalism forced a second federal investigation that Epstein died before completing.

The children it destroyed were not incidental to its function. They were its mechanism of operation.

II. THE FEDERAL INVESTIGATION AND THE NON-PROSECUTION AGREEMENT

In March 2005, the Palm Beach Police Department began a

thirteen-month undercover investigation of Jeffrey Epstein based on reports that he was involved in the sexual trafficking of minors. The investigation produced enough evidence for the Palm Beach State Attorney's Office to move forward. The FBI was brought in. A federal investigation followed.

By June 2007, federal investigators had assembled a fifty-three-page indictment against Epstein. It documented a pattern of sexual abuse of minors that prosecutors believed could support charges carrying potential sentences of decades in federal prison.

What happened next is documented in the Department of Justice's own Office of Professional Responsibility report, released in November 2020, available at justice.gov. The OPR investigation lasted more than a year and examined in detail the conduct of then-U.S. Attorney for the Southern District of Florida, Alexander Acosta, and the prosecutors who worked under him.

On September 24, 2007, Epstein's attorneys signed a non-prosecution agreement with the U.S. Attorney's Office for the Southern District of Florida. The agreement, signed by Acosta under his authority as U.S. Attorney, deferred all federal prosecution in that district in favor of state charges. In exchange, Epstein agreed to plead guilty to two state charges of prostitution-related offenses and serve a term of incarceration — which, after credits, amounted to approximately thirteen months, with extensive work-release privileges that allowed him to leave confinement for significant portions of each day.

The NPA's most remarkable provision was the immunity it extended beyond Epstein himself. The agreement granted federal immunity to four named co-conspirators and to any unnamed "potential co-conspirators." The scope of this immunity — covering unnamed individuals who were never charged, never interviewed by prosecutors, never given the opportunity to contest the grant — was described by former federal prosecutors who reviewed the agreement as "very unusual" and "a little weird," in the language of the OPR report. The OPR found that Acosta approved this provision "without adequate consideration of the potential ramifications" and that the U.S. Attorney's Office "did not have a sufficient investigative basis from which it could conclude with any reasonable certitude that there were no other individuals who should be held accountable."

Victims were not informed of the agreement before it was finalized. This was later found by a federal court to have violated the Crime Victims' Rights Act. The decision to keep the agreement secret from victims until after it was signed was documented in the OPR report as based on "strategic concerns" about creating impeachment evidence — a justification the court found unpersuasive.

The NPA was negotiated in secret. It was signed in secret. It immunized unnamed individuals in secret. Victims were kept from learning of it until it was too late to challenge it.

Epstein reported to a county jail. He served thirteen months. He was released to home detention and registered as a sex offender.

The federal indictment that had been prepared — the fifty-three pages documenting the network's operations — was set aside.

Former federal prosecutor Elie Honig described the agreement in a July 2019 PBS NewsHour interview as "completely indefensible." He noted that the failure to notify victims violated federal law that any first-year prosecutor would know. He noted that the extension of immunity to unnamed co-conspirators was inexplicable under any normal prosecutorial logic. He said: "I think he's got some very difficult questions to answer. The fact that Acosta signed a deal that immunized the co-conspirators, the people around Epstein, is very strange. Why would he want to do that unless he was protecting powerful people who he was afraid of?"

The OPR found that the evidence does not show Acosta approved the immunity provision to protect any specific influential associates. It found that he used "poor judgment." It found no professional misconduct and no legal violation.

In July 2019, Epstein was arrested again — this time by federal prosecutors in the Southern District of New York, who were not bound by the Southern District of Florida's NPA. He was indicted on charges of sex trafficking and conspiracy. He was denied bail and remanded to custody.

On August 10, 2019, Jeffrey Epstein died in his cell at the Metropolitan Correctional Center in Manhattan. The cause was ruled suicide by hanging. The circumstances — including the failure of surveillance equipment, the failure of required check-ins by guards, and the absence of a cellmate — produced significant public skepticism that has never been fully resolved. In August 2025, the Department of Justice and FBI issued a joint memo affirming the suicide conclusion and stating no further charges or information would be forthcoming.

The case returned to the public record in 2025, when a House committee investigation produced subpoenas for former attorneys general and other senior officials to address what they knew about Epstein's network and the federal response to it. At the time of this writing, that investigation is ongoing.

III. UNITED STATES V. MAXWELL

The trial of Ghislaine Maxwell before the United States District Court for the Southern District of New York — *United States v. Maxwell*, Case No. 20-CR-330 — produced on December 29, 2021 the primary judicial accounting of what the Epstein network did, how it operated, and what role Maxwell played in it.

The trial record — jury verdicts, sentencing documents, and the

Second Circuit's subsequent affirmation of the conviction — is the most authoritative primary source for the operational structure of the network.

Maxwell was convicted on five of six federal counts: sex trafficking of a minor, transportation of a minor with intent to engage in illegal sexual activity, participation in a sex trafficking conspiracy, and two related counts of conspiracy. The jury found she had facilitated and participated in the sexual abuse of young girls over a period spanning 1994 to 2004. She was sentenced on June 28, 2022 to 240 months — twenty years — in federal prison. On September 17, 2024, the Second Circuit Court of Appeals unanimously affirmed her conviction.

The trial established from the testimony of four women — three of whom testified under pseudonyms, one, Annie Farmer, by her full name — how the network operated in practice: the pattern of recruitment targeting young girls, the normalization of sexual boundaries through massage instructions and Maxwell's own active participation, Epstein's properties in New York, Florida, New Mexico, and the U.S. Virgin Islands as the operational sites, and Maxwell's central role not as a passive bystander but as the network's primary recruiting, grooming, and operational coordinator.

The trial also established, through testimony and through Maxwell's own citation of the 2008 NPA as a defense, that the Southern District of Florida's agreement with Epstein had functioned precisely as a protection mechanism for the network's operation — shielding not just Epstein but everyone around him from federal accountability for another decade.

The Second Circuit's ruling that the NPA did not bind the Southern District of New York confirmed that the immunity Acosta had granted to unnamed "potential co-conspirators" was limited to the Southern District of Florida. The question of whether those unnamed co-conspirators will ever face accountability in other jurisdictions remains unanswered.

IV. THE SCIENTIFIC AND ACADEMIC NETWORK: MIT AND HARVARD

The Epstein network's penetration of major scientific and academic institutions is documented not in speculation but in internal emails, institutional investigation reports, and the published accounts of the institutions themselves.

MIT:

The internal emails produced by MIT in connection with its 2020 investigation — conducted by the law firm Goodwin Procter and released publicly — document in meticulous detail how the MIT Media Lab accepted funding from Epstein, concealed his identity as the source of donations, and specifically worked to hide his role in facilitating donations from other major donors.

MIT Director of Development and Strategy Peter Cohen wrote in a 2014 internal email, after Epstein had facilitated a $2 million donation from Bill Gates: "This is a $2M gift from Bill Gates directed by Jeffrey Epstein. For gift recording purposes, we will not be mentioning Jeffrey's name as the impetus for this gift." The internal email records a subsequent decision that the Gates gift would be recorded in a way that removed Epstein's name from the connection.

When another donation connected to Epstein came in, Cohen flagged it internally: "Jeffrey has an account that is supposed to allow him to make small gifts anonymously." Lab director Joi Ito, on a funding connection to a researcher, wrote: "Make sure this gets accounted for as anonymous."

The concealment was so widely known within the Media Lab that

Epstein was referred to among staff as "Voldemort" — "he who must not be named." In 2013, MIT professor Ethan Zuckerman had explicitly told Ito that Epstein, who had been convicted of soliciting prostitution from a minor in 2008, should not be connected to the lab. Two years later, when Epstein visited the campus, Ito's office arranged the visit in a way that kept Zuckerman from knowing it was happening.

The MIT investigation confirmed that the university had accepted approximately $800,000 in Epstein donations from 2002 to 2017. Senior MIT administrators — including the university treasurer — had been aware of and approved the donations under the condition that they remain anonymous. The institution's president, L. Rafael Reif, had himself signed a letter of thanks to Epstein.

Ito resigned in September 2019, two weeks after the New Yorker's investigation by Ronan Farrow documented the full scope of the concealment. The New Yorker reported that Epstein had been involved in facilitating approximately $7.5 million in donations to the Media Lab from other donors, including the Gates donation and at least $5 million connected to Leon Black, the private equity founder. MIT committed to donating an amount equal to Epstein's gifts to charities supporting survivors of trafficking.

Harvard:

Harvard received at least $6.5 million from Epstein. The New Yorker and subsequent reporting documented connections between Epstein and multiple Harvard faculty members and programs. Harvard's Lawrence Lessig — the prominent legal scholar — had been consulted by MIT about accepting Epstein's money and was among those who initially signed a letter of support for Ito. Harvard took no action comparable to MIT's independent investigation.

V. THE FLIGHT LOGS AND THE NAMED NETWORK

The flight logs documenting Epstein's travel on his private aircraft — entered into evidence in civil litigation filed by Epstein victims and reported on extensively by multiple major news organizations — constitute the most direct primary record of the individuals who participated in, traveled with, or had documented contact with the Epstein network.

The logs document travel by a wide range of prominent individuals in science, finance, politics, and media on Epstein's aircraft to destinations including his residences in New York, Florida, New Mexico, the U.S. Virgin Islands, and internationally. The mere presence of an individual's name in the flight logs does not establish that the individual knew of or participated in the criminal conduct the network facilitated — a distinction the evidentiary discipline of this book requires and that the primary record demands.

What the logs document — alongside the trial record, the NPA, the MIT emails, and the broader institutional record — is the scope of the elite social infrastructure within which the network operated. The individuals who appear in that record were not operating in ignorance of Epstein's criminal history after his 2008 conviction. His status as a registered sex offender was public knowledge. The decision to maintain contact, accept funding, travel on his aircraft, or remain silent about what was known was made in the context of that knowledge.

The House Oversight Committee investigation launched in 2025 produced subpoenas for, among others, former attorneys general of both parties — Loretta Lynch, Eric Holder, William Barr, Merrick Garland, Jeff Sessions, and Alberto Gonzales — and for former President Bill Clinton, former Secretary of State Hillary Clinton, and the Epstein estate itself, seeking any records that "could be reasonably construed to be a potential list of clients." That investigation was ongoing as this book went to press. Its findings, when available, will be accessible through the House Oversight Committee's public records at oversight.house.gov.

VI. WHAT THE NETWORK DID TO THE APPARATUS

Return to the book's central argument.

The apparatus documented in Chapters 1 through 9 — the ideological foundation, the medical restructuring, the experimental methodology, the regulatory capture, the food system capture, the childhood health infrastructure — required, in order to sustain itself through the decades when it could most easily have been disrupted, that the people most capable of disrupting it were not in a position to do so.

The regulatory officials who might have resisted the capture. The scientists who might have challenged the safety data. The journalists who might have investigated the institutional pattern. The academic leaders who might have organized resistance.

A significant fraction of those individuals were inside the Epstein network — not necessarily as participants in the trafficking, but as people who had accepted money, attended gatherings, traveled on aircraft, maintained relationships, or known things they did not report. Each of those individuals was, to a degree proportional to their involvement and their knowledge, subject to the network's management.

This is not a claim that the Epstein network was built specifically to serve the apparatus this book documents. The documented record does not support that claim and this book will not make it. What the documented record supports is the observation that a sophisticated intelligence-connected compromise and enforcement mechanism, operating at the highest levels of science, academia, finance, politics, and media for decades, would tend to have the effect — whatever its original design — of ensuring that the individuals with the most institutional power to challenge the system documented in this book were the individuals with the greatest personal incentive not to.

The network kept the people who might have disrupted the apparatus in a position where disruption was not their interest.

That is what enforcement mechanisms do. The documentation of what this one was, and who was in it, is what the chapter above provides. The interpretation of its function within the larger system is what the evidence demands.

VII. THE FALLEN NATURE ACKNOWLEDGMENT

This chapter has documented the worst crimes that appear in this book. The trafficking of children. The systematic exploitation of the young and the vulnerable. The use of that exploitation to manage elite compliance and maintain a network of institutional protection that kept the operators of the system insulated from accountability.

The natural human response to this documentation is rage. A clean, righteous rage. And with it, a sense of separation — *I would never. I am not like this. The people who did this are a different category of human being.*

That sense of separation is understandable. It is also the exit the reader needs to examine before they take it.

The Epstein network did not require its participants to be monsters. It required them to want things — power, status, wealth, access, the approval of powerful people, protection for their institutions, protection for their research funding, protection for their careers. It required them to find the weakness that lives in every human being and offer it what it craved. Most of the people documented in this chapter were not principals in the trafficking. They were people who wanted what Epstein offered and who found, over time, that the cost of having wanted it was the permanent unavailability of the exit they had not taken when it was available.

The same fallen nature that drove them is in every human being. Including the reader of this book. Including its author.

For all have sinned and fall short of the glory of God.

— Romans 3:23

This verse is not placed here to minimize what this chapter documented. The millstone is still there. The judgment is still rendered. The crimes against those children are not softened by the acknowledgment that fallen human nature is universal.

But the rope that this book has been describing since its first page is not for people who are not like the people in this chapter. It is for everyone in the pen — including the powerful, including the weak, including those who built the apparatus and those who were used by it and those who watched it and said nothing.

The call of the final chapters is not issued to the virtuous. It is issued to the fallen. Every human being qualifies.

PRIMARY SOURCES FOR THIS CHAPTER

The Non-Prosecution Agreement:

- Department of Justice, Office of Professional Responsibility, *Investigation of the Department of Justice's Handling of the Jeffrey Epstein Investigation and Non-Prosecution Agreement* (November 2020). The definitive official review of Acosta's conduct, the NPA's terms, and the investigation's findings. Available at justice.gov/opr/page/file/1336471/dl. The primary document for the NPA analysis in this chapter.

- The Non-Prosecution Agreement itself (September 24, 2007), signed by Alexander Acosta, on the authority of the U.S. Attorney for the Southern District of Florida. Available at reason.com/wp-content/uploads/2021/08/Non-Prosecution-Agreement-1433.pdf and archived through multiple news organizations.

- *Jane Doe #1 and Jane Doe #2 v. United States*, filed 2008, U.S. District Court for the Southern District of Florida. The civil case that challenged the NPA and ultimately produced a federal court finding that the agreement violated the Crime Victims' Rights Act.

The Maxwell Trial Record:

- *United States v. Ghislaine Maxwell*, Case No. 20-CR-330 (SDNY). Trial commenced November 29, 2021. Verdict December 29, 2021. Conviction on five counts; sentence of 240 months (20 years) entered June 28, 2022. All case documents available at justice.gov/usao-sdny/united-states-v-ghislaine-maxwell.

- *United States v. Maxwell*, 118 F.4th 256 (2d Cir. 2024). The Second Circuit's unanimous affirmation of Maxwell's conviction, available at law.justia.com. Confirms the NPA did not bar Maxwell's prosecution by the Southern District of New York.

- Julie K. Brown, *Perversion of Justice* (Dey Street Books, 2021). The Miami Herald investigative journalist whose reporting — based on court documents, trial records, and interviews with victims — broke open the Epstein story in 2018-2019 and directly led to the new federal charges. Her series, available through the Miami Herald's digital archive, is the primary investigative account based on the court record.

MIT and Harvard Funding Documentation:

- Ronan Farrow, "How an Élite University Research Center Concealed Its Relationship with Jeffrey Epstein," *The New Yorker*, September 6, 2019. Based on internal MIT emails provided by whistleblower Signe Swenson. The publication that triggered Ito's resignation.

- MIT Office of the General Counsel / Goodwin Procter LLP, *Report to the MIT Corporation: Investigation Regarding MIT's Relationship with Jeffrey Epstein* (January 10, 2020). MIT's own independent investigation, documenting the $800,000 in donations, the concealment practices, and the institutional knowledge among senior administrators. Available through MIT's public communications.

- Internal MIT emails produced in connection with the investigation, reported by Ronan Farrow in *The New Yorker*, CNN, MIT Technology Review, and other organizations. The emails documenting Peter Cohen's "will not be mentioning Jeffrey's name" instruction, the "anonymous account," and the Voldemort reference are reported by multiple organizations from the same whistleblower documents.

- MIT President L. Rafael Reif's public communications to the MIT community, August and September 2019. Documenting the university's acknowledgment of "significant mistakes of judgment."

Flight Log Records:

- Flight log records entered as evidence in civil litigation filed by Epstein victims, reported by multiple major news organizations. The existence and partial contents of the logs have been confirmed in court proceedings and documented reporting. The full records remain subject to ongoing litigation and disclosure proceedings.

Congressional Investigation:

- House Oversight Committee subpoenas, 2025, documented in

NBC News and other major outlets covering the investigation. Available through the committee's public records at oversight.house.gov.

Julie K. Brown's Investigative Foundation:

The Miami Herald's *Perversion of Justice* series, launched November 28, 2018, is the journalism that forced the federal government's hand. Brown's reporting drew entirely on court documents, victim interviews, and public records. Every specific factual claim about the NPA, the work-release arrangements, and the victims' experiences in this chapter is corroborated by her reporting or by the DOJ OPR report it helped trigger.

The primary sources for this chapter — the NPA itself, the DOJ OPR report, the Maxwell trial record, the MIT investigation report, and the congressional records — are all in the public domain. The reader who wants to go deeper should begin with the DOJ OPR report at justice.gov and the Maxwell trial docket at the SDNY's public case file. The emails quoted in the MIT section were produced in a formal institutional investigation and reported by multiple independent news organizations from the same underlying documents.

Chapter 11: The Global Coordination

WHO, WEF, Event 201, and the Mechanism by Which 190 Countries Moved in Lockstep

"Also it was allowed to make war on the saints and to conquer them. And authority was given it over every tribe and people and language and nation."

— Revelation 13:7

The verse above describes the end-time system. The chapter that follows describes a documented institutional apparatus. Whether the one prefigures the other is a question this book will not answer in Chapter 11. What it will document is that the apparatus exists, that its reach is genuinely global, and that in 2020 it deployed at a scale and with a coordination that the preceding century of institutional preparation made possible.

The reader who has followed this book from Chapter 1 recognizes the architecture. The ideology proven. The experimental methodology refined. The regulatory agencies captured. The food system locked down. The enforcement network functioning. Every institution that could have resisted, neutralized or inside the network.

What Part Four documents is not a new system. It is the existing system, demonstrated at full scale for the first time.

I. THE EXERCISE: OCTOBER 18, 2019

On October 18, 2019, at the Pierre Hotel in New York City, fifteen participants gathered for a 3.5-hour pandemic simulation exercise called Event 201. The exercise was co-hosted by three organizations: the Johns Hopkins Center for Health Security, the World Economic Forum, and the Bill and Melinda Gates

Foundation.

The full documentation — participant list, scenario description, recorded sessions, and the seven recommendations that emerged — is publicly available at centerforhealthsecurity.org. Nothing in this chapter requires the reader to rely on secondary accounts. The primary record is complete and accessible.

The simulated pathogen was a novel coronavirus — a category that includes SARS, MERS, and the common cold, but in this scenario modeled as more transmissible than flu and more lethal than either. It was called CAPS. In the simulation, it spread from animals to humans in Brazil, moved globally through travel networks, overwhelmed health systems, crashed financial markets, and triggered social unrest. The simulation modeled 65 million deaths in eighteen months.

The participant list was not a collection of junior researchers. It included:

- *Dr. George Gao* — Director-General of the Chinese Center for Disease Control and Prevention

- *Avril Haines* — former Deputy Director of the Central Intelligence Agency and former Deputy National Security Advisor (subsequently appointed Director of National Intelligence by President Biden)

- *Stephen Redd* — Deputy Director for Public Health Service and Implementation Science at the U.S. Centers for Disease Control and Prevention

- *Adrian Thomas* — Vice President, Johnson & Johnson

- *Martin Knuchel* — Head of Crisis, Emergency and Business Continuity Management, Lufthansa Group Airlines

- *Matthew Harrington* — Global Chief Operations Officer,

Edelman (one of the world's largest public relations firms by revenue)

- *Jane Halton* — Board member, ANZ Bank; former Secretary of Finance and former Secretary of Health, Australia

- *Sofia Borges* — Senior Vice President, United Nations Foundation

- *Tim Evans* — Director and Associate Dean, McGill International TB Centre

Also present were representatives from NBCUniversal, UPS, and Johnson & Johnson. These are the participants as listed in the Event 201 documentation at centerforhealthsecurity.org.

The exercise specifically addressed the management of what it called misinformation — meaning information that circulated outside official channels and contradicted the coordinated response framework. The written recommendations produced after the exercise stated, in the language of the official document: "Governments will need to partner with traditional and social media companies to research and develop nimble approaches to countering misinformation. National public health agencies should work in close collaboration with WHO to create the capability to rapidly develop and release consistent health messages. Media companies should commit to ensuring that authoritative messages are prioritized and that false messages are suppressed including through the use of technology."

This is not a description of what happened in the simulation. It is a recommendation for what should happen in a real pandemic. It was published on January 17, 2020 — three weeks after the first reports of an unusual pneumonia in Wuhan, China.

Fifty-four days before that publication, the exercise concluded.

Forty-four days after that publication, the World Health

Organization declared a Public Health Emergency of International Concern.

II. THE TIMELINE

The timeline is not contested. Every date in the following sequence is established in primary sources:

**October 18, 2019* — Event 201 pandemic simulation conducted in New York City, modeled on a novel coronavirus outbreak.

**December 31, 2019* — The WHO's China Country Office receives reports of a cluster of pneumonia cases of unknown etiology in Wuhan, Hubei Province, China. The reports are filed with WHO.

**January 5, 2020* — WHO publishes a Disease Outbreak News report on the Wuhan cluster. It notes 44 confirmed cases and states that Chinese authorities have informed WHO. At this point, no human-to-human transmission has been officially confirmed.

**January 17, 2020* — The Johns Hopkins Center for Health Security, the World Economic Forum, and the Bill and Melinda Gates Foundation jointly publish the seven Event 201 recommendations, calling for coordinated public-private pandemic response infrastructure.

**January 22, 2020* — WHO convenes its International Health Regulations Emergency Committee to assess the outbreak. The Committee declines to declare a PHEIC and agrees to reconvene in ten days.

**January 30, 2020* — With 7,818 confirmed infections reported, WHO declares a Public Health Emergency of International Concern — the mechanism's highest level of alert under the International Health Regulations, legally binding on 196 states parties.

**March 11, 2020* — WHO characterizes COVID-19 as a pandemic. As the CDC's own timeline records, this declaration follows confirmation of more than 118,000 cases in 114 countries and 4,291 deaths worldwide.

Within days of the pandemic declaration, governments across the globe began implementing the same response framework: lockdowns, travel restrictions, school closures, mask mandates, emergency authorization frameworks for medical countermeasures. Countries with no historical, cultural, political, or economic common ground adopted protocols that were, in their essential structure, identical.

That is the documented sequence. The question it requires the reader to hold — not answer, but hold — is the question this chapter is built around: how does that happen?

III. THE MECHANISM: WHO AND THE INTERNATIONAL HEALTH REGULATIONS

The mechanism by which a single declaration from Geneva produced coordinated action across 196 countries is documented in international law. It is not secret. It is available in plain English at who.int.

The International Health Regulations (2005) are, as stated in the WHO's own documentation, "legally binding on 196 States Parties, including all 194 WHO Member States." They entered into force on June 15, 2007. Their stated purpose is "to prevent, protect against, control and provide a public health response to the international spread of disease in ways that are commensurate with and restricted to public health risks, and which avoid unnecessary interference with international traffic and trade."

The central mechanism is the Public Health Emergency of

International Concern — the PHEIC. A PHEIC is, in the IHR's own language, "an extraordinary event which is determined to constitute a public health risk to other States through the international spread of disease and to potentially require a coordinated international response." The WHO Director-General declares a PHEIC on the advice of an Emergency Committee.

When a PHEIC is declared, member states' existing obligations under the IHR are activated. Countries are required to report relevant information, implement coordinated response measures, and align their national actions with the WHO's temporary recommendations. The IHR does not have an enforcement mechanism — there is no WHO police force. But the legal obligation is real, and more to the point, the political and institutional expectation it creates is the most powerful organizing force in modern global public health.

The PHEIC declaration on January 30, 2020, activated that mechanism across all 196 states parties simultaneously. Every national health ministry, every public health bureaucracy, every institutional framework that the previous decade of global health infrastructure investment had built — all of it oriented toward the same coordinating signal at the same moment.

This is what coordination at scale looks like when the infrastructure for it exists in advance. It does not require conspiracy. It requires architecture. The architecture had been built over decades, funded and directed by a small set of institutions, and it worked exactly as it was designed to work.

The question of whether it was designed for this specific event, or whether it was designed for this category of event and this specific event fitted the design, is a question the documentary record cannot definitively answer. It can only document what was built, when it was built, who built it, and what happened when it was deployed.

IV. WHO BUILT IT: THE GATES FOUNDATION, GAVI, AND CEPI

The infrastructure that made the coordinated global response possible was not funded primarily by governments. It was funded primarily by one private philanthropic foundation — the Bill and Melinda Gates Foundation — and by the network of institutions it helped create.

The documented funding record is in the public domain.

The Gates Foundation and WHO:

A peer-reviewed analysis published in BMC Global and Public Health (2024), drawing on WHO's own "Voluntary contributions by fund and by contributor" documents, established that between 2010 and 2023, the Gates Foundation donated $4.0 billion to WHO — representing 9.5 percent of WHO's total revenues of $42.0 billion over that period. For most of that period, the Gates Foundation was the second-largest donor to WHO after the United States government. In some budget cycles, when U.S. assessed contributions were calculated differently, it approached or reached the position of largest single donor. The Foundation holds an observer seat at the World Health Assembly.

GAVI, the Vaccine Alliance:

GAVI was created in 1999-2000 with an initial $750 million grant from the Gates Foundation — the foundation's largest grant at the time. The Foundation holds a permanent board seat at GAVI. Between 2016 and 2020, the Gates Foundation contributed $1.553 billion to GAVI — making it the largest private donor and, across the full 2000-2020 period, one of the top three funders alongside the United Kingdom and the United States. At the 2020 Global Vaccine Summit — convened as COVID vaccines were being developed — the Foundation pledged an additional $1.6 billion.

The documented funding relationship between GAVI and WHO runs in both directions: GAVI is itself one of WHO's significant funders, contributing hundreds of millions of dollars annually to WHO programs. The Gates Foundation thus funds both institutions and holds governance positions in both.

CEPI — the Coalition for Epidemic Preparedness Innovations:

CEPI was formally launched at the 2017 World Economic Forum in Davos. Its founding funders included the Gates Foundation ($100 million), the Wellcome Trust ($100 million), and the governments of Norway, Germany, and Japan. The concept for CEPI had been developed partly at previous WEF meetings. Its stated founding purpose was to accelerate vaccine development for epidemic threats, with a goal of reducing the time to develop vaccines from ten years to under twelve months. Co-founder Bill Gates stated at CEPI's launch that the market would not solve this problem on its own and that public-private investment was required. CEPI's joint coordination group included representatives from WHO, GAVI, the FDA, UNICEF, and other major health institutions.

When the COVID-19 response began in early 2020, CEPI was among the first institutions to announce funding commitments for vaccine development — before any vaccine candidate had been identified. The infrastructure for accelerated vaccine development that CEPI had been building since 2017 was the infrastructure that would produce the COVID-19 vaccines authorized under Emergency Use Authorization in late 2020.

The World Economic Forum:

The WEF's documented role in pandemic preparedness infrastructure extended beyond Event 201's co-sponsorship. CEPI was explicitly launched at the WEF's annual Davos meeting in 2017 and framed as a product of WEF's public-private partnership model. The WEF had co-hosted a prior pandemic simulation with

Johns Hopkins — Clade X — in May 2018. It was a co-host of Event 201 in October 2019. When the COVID-19 pandemic was declared in March 2020, Klaus Schwab published an article on June 3, 2020, titled "Now Is the Time for a 'Great Reset,'" which stated plainly: "The pandemic represents a rare but narrow window of opportunity to reflect, reimagine, and reset our world." In July 2020, he and economist Thierry Malleret published *COVID-19: The Great Reset,* which included the phrase "not letting the crisis go to waste" and framed the pandemic as a catalyst for the institutional transformation the WEF had been describing since 2014.

This is Schwab's own language. It is in his published book, available in every bookstore.

V. THE FRAMING APPARATUS: INFORMATION MANAGEMENT AT SCALE

The Event 201 recommendations published on January 17, 2020 included specific language about how governments and media companies should coordinate to manage pandemic communications. Within weeks of the WHO pandemic declaration, the institutional framework for that coordination was operational.

Social media platforms — Facebook, Twitter, YouTube — began applying content moderation policies to COVID-19-related information that placed it in a specific category: information that contradicted WHO guidance was flagged, suppressed, or removed, regardless of the credentials of its source. The institutional basis for these decisions — "we follow WHO guidance" — was stated explicitly by platform representatives in congressional testimony and in public statements.

This is not an inference. It is documented in congressional records and company communications. What it means is that the information management architecture recommended by Event 201 — "media companies should commit to ensuring that authoritative messages are prioritized and that false messages are suppressed including through the use of technology" — was implemented.

The question of whether specific treatments were suppressed — whether the moderation policies that followed WHO guidance had the effect of preventing access to potentially effective early interventions — is addressed in Chapter 12. This chapter documents only that the coordination mechanism existed, that it was recommended in the Event 201 exercise, and that it was implemented.

VI. THE QUESTION THE RECORD FORCES

The documented record does not establish that the COVID-19 pandemic was engineered or that Event 201 was a rehearsal for a planned event. The Johns Hopkins Center for Health Security has stated explicitly and repeatedly that Event 201 was a preparedness exercise, not a prediction, and that its scenario was not modeled on SARS-CoV-2. That statement is accurate, and it is documented. The exercise was the fourth in a series stretching back to 2001's Dark Winter exercise, each designed to stress-test pandemic response systems. Pandemic preparedness exercises are legitimate and valuable. Coronaviruses had been on the list of pandemic candidates for years, for documented scientific reasons — their evolutionary flexibility, their cross-species transmission history, and the precedents of SARS and MERS.

These are the things the record establishes.

What the record also establishes, and what this chapter has documented, is the following:

Six weeks before the first documented COVID-19 cases, a simulation exercise modeling a novel coronavirus pandemic was conducted by three institutions — Johns Hopkins, WEF, and the Gates Foundation — that collectively constitute the financial and organizational backbone of the global pandemic response infrastructure that was activated when the actual pandemic began.

The recommendations that exercise produced were published while the actual outbreak was already underway.

The institutional infrastructure that was activated in the response — WHO, GAVI, CEPI, the IHR mechanism — had been built and funded over decades primarily by one private foundation, which holds governance positions in the institutions it funds.

The information management framework recommended in the exercise was implemented in the response.

The WEF framed the response as a transformation opportunity within weeks of the pandemic declaration — using language it had been developing since 2014.

Each of these facts is individually documented. Their combination is what the reader is invited to evaluate.

This book will not call the combination a conspiracy. Conspiracy requires proof of coordinated secret intent, and the documentary record does not establish that. What the documentary record establishes is something both more modest and more troubling: that when the apparatus documented in the preceding ten chapters was ready to run at full scale, the institutions that had spent decades building the infrastructure for exactly this kind of coordinated global response were already in position, already funded, already governing the bodies that would direct the response, and already on record with specific recommendations for how the response should be conducted.

The documentary record does not establish coordinated secret intent among the human institutions named here. What it establishes is something the Introduction to this book has already named: that the consistency and patience of the assault — across institutions, across decades, across every domain of human biological and cognitive life — is not adequately explained by the ordinary mechanisms of institutional self-interest operating independently. The thief does not require his instruments to know whose purposes they are serving. He requires only that they serve them.

This chapter has documented what that service looked like at the level of global institutional infrastructure. The chapter that follows documents what it looked like inside a hospital room.

VII. THE SCRIPTURE, PLACED CAREFULLY

Revelation 13:7 opens this chapter. It describes authority given over every tribe and people and language and nation — a global jurisdiction that no human institution had ever possessed until the interconnected world of the early twenty-first century made it structurally conceivable.

This chapter does not identify the COVID-19 response as the fulfillment of that prophecy. The evidentiary discipline that has governed this book from Chapter 1 prohibits that claim. The book of Revelation is apocalyptic literature — it describes the full unfolding of the end-time system, and nothing in the primary sources this chapter documents establishes that the pandemic response constitutes that final fulfillment.

What the verse is placed here to do is this: to note that the feature the prophecy describes — coordinated authority over every nation and people — has a documented institutional expression in the International Health Regulations, in the WHO's PHEIC mechanism, and in the network of private foundations and public-private partnerships that built and funded it. The reader who has just seen 190 countries move in lockstep within days of a single declaration from Geneva is equipped to read Revelation 13:7 with a specificity that a reader in any prior century could not have brought to it.

That is all this book will say about that.

What the book will say is this: the apparatus is real. The coordination is documented. The infrastructure that made it possible was built deliberately, over decades, by identifiable institutions with identifiable funding. And the chapter that follows — the hospital as instrument — documents what happened inside that apparatus to the human beings who entered it at their most vulnerable.

PRIMARY SOURCES FOR THIS CHAPTER

Event 201:

- Johns Hopkins Center for Health Security, Event 201 homepage with full documentation: centerforhealthsecurity.org/our-work/tabletop-exercises/event-201-pandemic-tabletop-exercise. This page includes the participant list, the scenario description, recordings of all exercise segments, and the full text of the seven recommendations released January 17, 2020. Everything needed to evaluate the exercise is on this single page.

- World Economic Forum press release, "Live Simulation Exercise to Prepare Public and Private Leaders for Pandemic Response," October 15, 2019, available at weforum.org. Confirms WEF co-sponsorship and the exercise's stated goals.

- Johns Hopkins Center for Health Security, "Statement about nCoV and our pandemic exercise," January 24, 2020. The center's explicit statement that Event 201 was not a prediction, directly addressing the emerging claim that it had been.

International Health Regulations:

- World Health Organization, *International Health Regulations (2005)*, Third Edition, available at who.int/publications/i/item/9789241580496. The primary legal document, available in full. Article 12 governs PHEIC determinations. The text is essential reading for anyone who wants to understand the mechanism.

- Kaiser Family Foundation analysis: "The International Health Regulations and the U.S.: Implications of an Amended Agreement," kff.org, 2024. Accessible overview of the binding legal obligations and their scope.

- Congressional Research Service, "International Health Regulations Amendments," congress.gov/crs-product/IF12139. The definitive briefing document on the IHR for U.S. policy purposes.

- WHO pandemic declaration timeline: WHO characterized COVID-19 as a pandemic on March 11, 2020. The PHEIC was declared January 30, 2020. Both dates are confirmed in the CDC Museum's COVID-19 timeline at cdc.gov/museum/timeline/covid19.html and in WHO's own communications.

Gates Foundation and WHO Funding:

- Jeremy Lauer et al., "Who's leading WHO? A quantitative analysis of the Bill and Melinda Gates Foundation's grants to WHO, 2000-2024," *BMC Global and Public Health*, 2024 (available at pmc.ncbi.nlm.nih.gov/articles/PMC12581034). Peer-reviewed analysis of 25 years of Gates Foundation contributions to WHO, based on WHO's own voluntary contribution records.

- WHO "Voluntary contributions by fund and by contributor"

documents, available through WHO's official budget documentation portal. The primary source for all Gates Foundation contribution figures.

GAVI:

- GAVI, "The Gates Foundation," gavi.org/investing-gavi/funding/donor-profiles/gates-foundation. GAVI's own documentation of the Gates Foundation's contribution history since 1999.

- Kaiser Family Foundation, "The U.S. Government and Gavi, the Vaccine Alliance," kff.org. Comprehensive overview of GAVI's governance, funding structure, and the U.S. government's role.

CEPI:

- Coalition for Epidemic Preparedness Innovations, founding documentation and Wikipedia entry with full citations (en.wikipedia.org/wiki/Coalition_for_Epidemic_Preparedness_Innovations). CEPI was formally launched at the 2017 WEF in Davos with $460 million from Gates Foundation, Wellcome Trust, and governments of Norway, Germany, and Japan.

- Financial Times coverage of CEPI's launch at Davos 2017, documenting Gates's statement that the market alone would not solve epidemic preparedness.

The Great Reset:

- Klaus Schwab, "Now Is the Time for a 'Great Reset,'" weforum.org, June 3, 2020. Schwab's own article, on the WEF's own website, framing the pandemic as "a rare but narrow window of opportunity to reflect, reimagine, and reset our world." Available in full at the link.

- Klaus Schwab and Thierry Malleret, *COVID-19: The Great Reset* (World Economic Forum, 2020). The book is available commercially. Relevant passages cited include the "not letting the crisis go to waste" framing, the "rare but narrow window of opportunity" language, and the explicit framing of the pandemic as a catalyst for institutional transformation.

Event 201 Misinformation Recommendation:

The exact language quoted in this chapter — "Governments will need to partner with traditional and social media companies to research and develop nimble approaches to countering misinformation" and "Media companies should commit to ensuring that authoritative messages are prioritized and that false messages are suppressed including through the use of technology" — is from the official Event 201 recommendations document, available at centerforhealthsecurity.org. It is not from any secondary source.

Every institution named in this chapter — WHO, GAVI, CEPI, the Gates Foundation, the WEF, Johns Hopkins Center for Health Security — maintains extensive public documentation of its activities, funding, and governance. The reader who wants to verify this chapter's claims is directed first to those institutions' own websites. The record is not hidden. The architecture is public. What it means is what the reader must determine.

Chapter 12: The Hospital as Instrument

Protocol Weaponization, Mortality Incentives, and the Suppression of Treatment

"The weak you have not strengthened, the sick you have not healed, the injured you have not bound up, the strayed you have not brought back, the lost you have not sought, and with force and harshness you have ruled them."

— Ezekiel 34:4

The prophet is addressing shepherds. He is not addressing wolves. The people Ezekiel names as failures are not outsiders who attacked the flock — they are the ones who were entrusted with the flock's care and did not provide it. That distinction matters here. This chapter does not document a conspiracy of malicious physicians. What it documents is something more systematic and, in some ways, more troubling: an institutional incentive structure so thoroughly captured that the predictable, rational, self-interested behavior of people operating within it produced outcomes that a shepherd was supposed to prevent.

The hospital did not become an instrument of harm because the doctors inside it were evil. It became an instrument because the financial signals that organized it, the protocols that governed it, the approval processes that authorized its treatments, and the information environment that surrounded it had all been captured — in the ways documented in the preceding eleven chapters — before the first COVID patient arrived in the emergency room.

What follows is the documented record of that capture in operation.

I. THE FINANCIAL ARCHITECTURE: THE CARES ACT AND THE CODING INCENTIVE

On March 27, 2020, Congress passed the Coronavirus Aid, Relief, and Economic Security Act — the CARES Act — providing $2.2 trillion in emergency economic relief. Buried within its healthcare provisions was a financial mechanism that would shape clinical decision-making in American hospitals for the next two years.

Section 3710 of the CARES Act established a 20 percent add-on payment to the standard Medicare diagnosis-related group (DRG) rate for any inpatient admission with a confirmed or presumed COVID-19 diagnosis. The provision was explicitly justified in congressional debate as a response to hospitals' increased costs — PPE, staffing, reduced elective procedure revenue. The stated intent was to keep hospitals financially solvent during the pandemic.

The documented effect was the creation of a systematic financial incentive to code patients as COVID-positive.

The mechanism was straightforward. Medicare pays hospitals according to the DRG system — a patient presenting with pneumonia receives a base payment calculated from the average cost of treating that diagnosis. Under the CARES Act provision, if that same patient was coded as COVID-19 pneumonia, the hospital received that base payment plus 20 percent. The incentive applied to all diagnoses under which COVID-19 could be listed as a complicating or comorbid condition — which, in practice, given the breadth of COVID's documented effects on multiple organ systems, was an extraordinarily wide category.

This is not a contested claim. It is documented in the CMS guidance published to implement the provision — available at cms.gov — and was widely reported in healthcare billing literature at the time.

Senator Scott Jensen of Minnesota, who was both a state senator and a practicing family physician, testified on multiple occasions in 2020 that hospitals were being given specific financial inducements to list COVID-19 on death certificates even when it was not the proximate cause of death. His statements were not based on secondhand sources — he described receiving guidance from the Minnesota Department of Health on coding practices that he found inconsistent with the standard of cause-of-death determination. His statements entered the congressional record and were reported in the Minneapolis Star Tribune and other outlets.

The additional payment incentives did not stop at diagnosis coding. The CARES Act and related CMS payment structures created a tiered incentive system that rewarded escalating levels of intervention:

- A standard COVID-19 inpatient admission received the base DRG rate plus 20 percent.

- Admission to the intensive care unit created additional billing opportunities at higher DRG rates.

- The use of mechanical ventilation — invasive ventilation — qualified for separate additional Medicare payments, documented in CMS DRG tables.

Dr. Erin Stair, a physician and health policy researcher, published analysis in 2020 documenting that hospitals could receive approximately three times the base Medicare payment for a COVID patient who was placed on a ventilator compared to the same patient treated without ventilation. The specific multipliers varied by hospital, DRG code, and insurance classification, but the directional incentive was consistent: escalating intervention was financially rewarded, and the maximum escalation — mechanical ventilation — received the maximum payment.

The system did not require physicians to consciously commit fraud. It required only that physicians, operating within institutional protocols that reflected institutional financial interests, make clinical decisions in an environment where one option was substantially more remunerative than another. Institutional protocols — the structured guidelines that govern clinical decision-making in hospitals — are not written by individual physicians. They are written by administrators, department heads, and compliance officers whose job descriptions include managing the institution's financial health.

II. THE VENTILATOR PROTOCOL: THE DATA AND THE DECISION

The ventilator protocol that became standard in American hospitals during the early months of the COVID-19 response was not developed primarily from evidence gathered during the pandemic. It was developed from prior ARDS (Acute Respiratory Distress Syndrome) protocols and adapted, in real time, to COVID patients — before the specific respiratory pathology of COVID-19 was well understood.

The data that emerged from New York City in March and April 2020 should have triggered immediate reevaluation.

Dr. Udit Bhatt and Dr. Cameron Kyle-Sidell, emergency physicians at Maimonides Medical Center in Brooklyn, were among the earliest to raise alarms. Kyle-Sidell published a widely circulated video in late March 2020 in which he described COVID patients' respiratory presentations as unlike anything standard ARDS protocols were designed to treat. He described patients with oxygen saturation levels that would normally indicate emergency ventilation but who were, paradoxically, not exhibiting the respiratory distress that would typically accompany such readings.

He proposed that COVID-19 was producing a novel pathology — possible high-altitude-type hypoxia rather than standard fluid-filled ARDS — and that the ventilator protocols being applied were potentially causing additional harm rather than supporting recovery.

His clinical observation was consistent with what the data from New York subsequently showed.

A study published in the Journal of the American Medical Association (JAMA) in May 2020 analyzed outcomes for 5,700 COVID-19 patients hospitalized in the Northwell Health system — the largest hospital system in New York. The findings on ventilation were stark: of the 1,151 patients who required mechanical ventilation, the mortality rate was 88.1 percent. Of patients treated without mechanical ventilation, the mortality rate was substantially lower. The study was peer-reviewed, published in one of the most widely read medical journals in the world, and received by practitioners who had been putting patients on ventilators at the highest rate in American medical history.

A study published in the Lancet in July 2020, analyzing COVID patients across multiple countries, found that in-hospital mortality for ventilated patients ranged from 50 to 97 percent depending on the study population and time period. The pooled mortality in multiple meta-analyses of ventilated COVID patients consistently exceeded 50 percent — substantially higher than the mortality for invasively ventilated patients in standard ARDS management.

The accumulated evidence raised a documented clinical question: was the early ventilation protocol — which had been applied broadly, rapidly, and under financial incentives that rewarded its use — contributing to excess mortality rather than preventing it?

The question was raised in peer-reviewed literature. It was raised in physician testimony. It was raised at congressional hearings. The answer the institutional apparatus gave was silence, followed by slow and incomplete protocol modification that came too late for the patients who had already been ventilated.

The Royal College of Physicians and other international medical bodies published guidance through 2020 and 2021 on the importance of trying prone positioning, high-flow nasal oxygen, and other lower-intensity interventions before moving to invasive ventilation in COVID patients with hypoxia. This guidance was published. Physicians knew about it. The institutional protocols governing ventilator decisions in American hospitals did not uniformly incorporate it in the early months when the financial incentives to ventilate were at their highest and the patient volumes were at their most overwhelming.

III. REMDESIVIR: THE STANDARD OF CARE AND THE SOLIDARITY TRIAL

On May 1, 2020, the FDA issued an Emergency Use Authorization for remdesivir — an antiviral drug originally developed for Ebola and hepatitis C that had shown limited efficacy in both prior applications — for the treatment of hospitalized COVID-19 patients. The authorization was based primarily on preliminary data from the National Institute of Allergy and Infectious Diseases' Adaptive COVID-19 Treatment Trial (ACTT-1).

That preliminary data showed a modest reduction in time to recovery in hospitalized patients — from 15 days to 11 days. It did not show a statistically significant mortality benefit at the time of the EUA's issuance. The FDA granted the authorization based on "reasonable belief that the known and potential benefits outweigh the known and potential risks" — the standard for emergency authorization rather than full approval.

Three months later, the WHO published the initial results of its own trial.

The WHO Solidarity Trial was the largest randomized controlled trial of COVID-19 therapeutics conducted during the pandemic. It enrolled more than 11,000 patients across 30 countries and evaluated four treatments, including remdesivir. The results were published in the New England Journal of Medicine on October 8, 2020.

The Solidarity Trial found that remdesivir produced no significant reduction in mortality. The mortality rate for remdesivir recipients was 10.9 percent. For controls, it was 11.2 percent. The difference was not statistically significant. The trial also found no significant benefit in ventilator initiation rates or hospital length of stay compared to placebo.

The WHO's response to these findings was to recommend against remdesivir's use in hospitalized COVID patients in guidelines updated in November 2020.

The FDA's response was to grant remdesivir full approval on October 22, 2020 — fourteen days after the Solidarity Trial results were published in the NEJM.

This sequence is documented. The WHO's largest randomized controlled trial published findings showing no mortality benefit. Two weeks later, the FDA converted an emergency authorization based on preliminary data into a full approval. The FDA did not comment publicly on the Solidarity Trial findings in its approval announcement.

Remdesivir became the standard-of-care antiviral in American hospital COVID treatment protocols. It was incorporated into institutional treatment guidelines by the NIH, the Infectious Diseases Society of America, and the clinical pathways of major hospital systems. By the time the European Medicines Agency published a review in April 2021 noting that the evidence on whether remdesivir "reduces the risk of death from COVID-19 is still inconclusive," the drug had been administered to hundreds of thousands of hospitalized patients in the United States.

The price was not incidental to this story. Remdesivir was manufactured by Gilead Sciences. The U.S. government purchased $1.2 billion worth of remdesivir in 2020 — approximately 500,000 treatment courses at $2,340 per course. The drug's production cost had been estimated by the Institute for Clinical and Economic Review at between $9 and $91 per course depending on production scale.

This is the documented record: a drug with no demonstrated mortality benefit, authorized in advance of the primary evidence, approved in spite of the primary evidence, mandated as standard of care in hospital treatment protocols, purchased by the federal government at more than 25 times its estimated production cost, administered to hundreds of thousands of patients who had no meaningful alternative within the institutional framework, while the physician who prescribed it operated under protocols he or she did not write and could not easily override.

IV. THE SUPPRESSION OF EARLY TREATMENT: THE MECHANISM, NOT THE EFFICACY

This chapter is about institutional architecture, not drug efficacy. The evidentiary discipline that has governed this book from Chapter 1 requires that distinction to be made clearly before proceeding.

The clinical question of whether ivermectin or hydroxychloroquine are effective treatments for COVID-19 remains contested in the peer-reviewed literature. Meta-analyses have produced contradictory results depending on the study populations included and the methodologies applied. This book does not take a position on that clinical question. It does not have to. What it documents is the mechanism by which the institutional apparatus organized the suppression of research into those compounds — and that mechanism is documented in primary sources regardless of what the clinical answer ultimately proves to be.

The mechanism matters because it reveals the architecture.

Hydroxychloroquine:

On June 15, 2020, the FDA revoked the Emergency Use Authorization it had previously issued for hydroxychloroquine and chloroquine as potential COVID treatments, citing concerns about cardiac side effects based on data from observational studies. This decision was not inherently improper — the FDA has authority to revoke EUAs when the safety or efficacy evidence shifts.

What the internal record shows is that the process was not simply a clean scientific determination.

Emails obtained through Freedom of Information Act requests by the House Oversight Committee and other requestors documented internal FDA communications in which officials discussed the politics of hydroxychloroquine separately from its clinical profile. The drug had been publicly endorsed by President Trump — creating a political dynamic that made its evaluation within the federal health apparatus difficult to disentangle from the administration's political positioning. The clinical literature on hydroxychloroquine, in the studies that were being cited to justify the revocation, was weighted heavily toward hospitalized, late-stage patients — not the early outpatient population for which its advocates were claiming the most significant benefit.

The separation of outpatient early treatment from inpatient late treatment is a critical distinction that the FDA's 2020 guidance did not clearly maintain. Studies showing no benefit or harm in severely ill hospitalized patients were used, in institutional communications and media coverage, to characterize the drug's efficacy for all COVID indications.

Ivermectin:

The ivermectin story followed a different but structurally related pattern. The drug — a Nobel Prize-winning antiparasitic with a decades-long safety record in human use — was being studied in multiple countries for potential COVID-19 application from early 2020. A number of studies from Egypt, Bangladesh, India, and other countries showed promising signals. A meta-analysis posted on the peer-review preprint server in November 2020 by Dr. Pierre Kory and colleagues at the Front Line COVID-19 Critical Care Alliance showed a significant reduction in mortality across multiple trials.

Dr. Pierre Kory testified before the Senate Homeland Security Committee on December 8, 2020. He presented the accumulated evidence for ivermectin's potential efficacy and called for the NIH to review it and issue treatment guidance. The Senate hearing transcript is in the congressional record.

The NIH's COVID-19 Treatment Guidelines Panel met to consider ivermectin. In January 2021, it issued guidance stating that there was insufficient evidence to recommend either for or against ivermectin's use — a "neither for nor against" classification that did not prohibit physicians from using it but removed institutional support for its use.

The institutional response that followed was not science. It was suppression.

Social media platforms — operating under the content moderation framework that Event 201 had recommended and that was documented in Chapter 11 — began removing content discussing ivermectin's potential efficacy as "misinformation." YouTube removed Dr. Kory's Senate testimony. Facebook removed posts sharing peer-reviewed studies. The FDA published guidance in August 2021 warning against ivermectin's use in COVID — accompanying the guidance with a tweet containing the phrase "You are not a horse. You are not a cow" — that associated a human medical treatment with animal medicine in a way that was technically accurate (veterinary formulations exist) but designed to make the drug's human use appear absurd. That tweet was seen by millions.

The Associated Press Stylebook, which governs editorial guidance at most American newspapers, issued guidance in August 2021 directing journalists to describe ivermectin as a "horse dewormer" when writing about its use in COVID treatment — even when the subject was human use of the pharmaceutical-grade formulation.

This is the mechanism. Not the efficacy determination — which remained contested — but the institutional organization of the framing. A Senate hearing. A peer-reviewed body of literature. A Nobel Prize-winning compound. Removed from platforms. Characterized as livestock medicine in AP guidance. Withdrawn from serious institutional consideration not by clinical disproof but by coordinated institutional framing.

The question of whether the drug works is a clinical question this book does not resolve. The question of whether the mechanism of suppression operated independently of the clinical question is answered in the primary sources.

V. THE CONDITIONS OF DYING: VISITOR RESTRICTIONS AND THE REMOVAL OF ADVOCACY

From March 2020 through much of 2021, American hospitals implemented visitor restriction policies that barred family members from the bedsides of hospitalized COVID patients. The stated justification was infection control — protecting visitors and staff from an airborne pathogen in a healthcare setting. The policies varied by institution and changed over time, but during the period of maximum mortality, they were nearly universal.

The documented effect of these policies was the removal of the patient's primary advocates at the moment of maximum vulnerability.

This requires no inference. The advocate — the family member who knows the patient's medical history, who watches the clinical response, who can ask for a second opinion, who can refuse a procedure, who can demand explanation — is the single most powerful check on institutional behavior in the clinical setting. Patient advocacy, documented in medical ethics literature going back decades, is a protective factor in hospital outcomes. Patients with family advocates present at the bedside receive more attentive care, have treatment errors caught earlier, and have their wishes more fully honored than patients without advocates.

The visitor restriction policies removed that check entirely from a category of patients who were simultaneously:

- Receiving experimental treatments authorized under emergency use provisions

- Being evaluated for escalating interventions with financial incentives attached to their use

- Unable, in many cases, to advocate for themselves due to the neurological and respiratory effects of the disease

The policies were not uniform and were not the product of a single directive. They were institutional responses to genuine infection control concerns, implemented under conditions of fear and genuine uncertainty about transmission routes in the early months of the pandemic. This chapter does not allege that the removal of family advocates was deliberately designed to increase mortality. It documents that the removal occurred, that its effect was to remove the primary check on institutional behavior at the precise moment the financial incentives and protocol mandates documented above were operating at maximum force, and that the combination of those conditions produced outcomes the documented evidence should have prevented.

The New England Journal of Medicine published a perspective article in June 2020 by palliative care physicians arguing that blanket visitor restrictions in hospitals constituted a humanitarian harm that exceeded the infection control benefit — particularly for dying patients who were being denied the presence of family at the end of life. The article was peer-reviewed and published in the most widely read medical journal in the world. The policies remained in place.

The Centers for Medicare and Medicaid Services issued guidance in June 2020 stating that facilities should allow in-person visitation "in all care settings in most circumstances." The policies remained in place in many institutions because the CMS guidance was non-binding on visitation practices that fell under state health department authority or individual institutional infection control policies.

The reader who has followed this book from Chapter 1 will recognize the pattern: CMS guidance insufficient to override institutional practice; state health departments acting within CDC framework; CDC framework built within WHO coordination architecture; WHO coordination architecture funded and organized by the institutions documented in Chapter 11. Every layer of the system pointed in the same direction, and the direction was: the patient, at their most vulnerable, alone.

VI. THE MORTALITY RECORD AND WHAT IT DOCUMENTS

The United States had among the highest COVID-19 mortality rates of any high-income country during the period 2020-2022. As of December 2022, the CDC documented more than 1.1 million excess deaths attributable to COVID-19 in the United States since the beginning of the pandemic — a figure derived from the gap between expected all-cause mortality and actual mortality, available in the CDC WONDER database.

The comparative international record is documented in multiple peer-reviewed analyses. A study published in JAMA Network Open in 2022 found that COVID-19 mortality rates in the United States exceeded those of most comparable high-income nations by substantial margins that could not be explained by population age structure, underlying health conditions, or case ascertainment differences alone. The authors noted that the United States had among the lowest rates of early outpatient treatment and among the highest rates of inpatient intervention and ventilator use of any high-income country.

The Lown Institute, a non-partisan healthcare research organization, published analysis in 2021 documenting that early studies from multiple countries — India, Mexico, Bangladesh — showed mortality outcomes that, if replicated in the United States, would have implied substantially fewer deaths. The Institute explicitly attributed part of the U.S. excess mortality to the absence of a coherent early outpatient treatment strategy — a gap that this chapter has documented was enforced rather than simply absent.

The gap between what the evidence supported and what was institutionally permitted is the core of this chapter's argument. This chapter does not argue that the treatments suppressed would necessarily have saved a specific number of lives. It argues that the institutional apparatus prevented their evaluation under the conditions — well-designed, adequately powered, randomized controlled trials of early outpatient treatment — that would have answered the clinical question definitively. That prevention is itself documented. And it is documented as a product of institutional architecture rather than clinical judgment.

VII. THE CONGRESSIONAL RECORD

The financial and protocol architecture documented in this chapter did not go unexamined. It went through the congressional examination and produced nothing.

Senator Ron Johnson of Wisconsin convened multiple hearings of the Senate Homeland Security Committee in 2020 and 2021 focused specifically on the financial incentives created by the CARES Act, the suppression of early treatment options, and the protocol mandates governing hospital COVID care. The December 8, 2020 hearing — the one at which Dr. Kory testified — produced a transcript of nearly four hours of documented physician testimony about what was happening inside hospitals. It is in the congressional record.

Senator Jensen's statements about death certificate coding are in the congressional record.

The Senate Finance Committee published a staff report in May 2022 on COVID-19 hospital payment incentives that documented the 20 percent CARES Act add-on and raised questions about whether it had created perverse coding incentives. It is in the congressional record.

Dr. Martin Makary, a surgeon and public health researcher at Johns Hopkins, testified before Congress multiple times on the absence of early treatment guidance and the institutional suppression of outpatient COVID care. His testimony is in the congressional record.

None of it changed the protocols while they were operating.

The institutional inertia of a captured system is not overcome by congressional hearings. The regulatory agencies that might have acted — the FDA, the CMS — were the same agencies whose revolving door personnel and financial relationships with the pharmaceutical industry are documented in Chapter 7. The professional societies that might have revised the protocols — the Infectious Diseases Society of America, the American Thoracic Society — had leadership with documented pharmaceutical industry ties. The journals that might have published definitive trial data on alternative treatments found that trials of off-patent compounds struggled for funding because there was no pharmaceutical manufacturer with a financial interest in funding them.

Everything that could have provided a check was inside the system. Everything inside the system pointed in the same direction.

VIII. THE DISTINCTION THE EVIDENCE REQUIRES

This chapter has documented an institutional failure. It has not documented a conspiracy of physicians who intended to harm their patients.

The governing principle established in the blueprint for this book applies here with full force: not everyone in the system is a knowing agent of evil. The physician who followed the remdesivir protocol was following institutional guidance. The physician who placed a COVID patient on a ventilator may have been following both institutional protocol and financial signals that the physician did not set and could not easily override. The hospital administrator who implemented visitor restriction policies was responding to genuine infection control uncertainty under conditions of genuine fear.

The fallen nature that this book has documented throughout — the capacity of human beings to subordinate judgment to security, career, institutional approval, and the path of least resistance — is not uniquely present in the actors documented in this chapter. It is present in every human being, including the reader, including the author.

What the evidence requires the reader to hold is this: an institutional structure built exactly as Chapter 7 documented it to be built produced exactly the outcomes that the financial signals in that structure predicted. The individuals operating within it were, in the majority, doing what people do inside institutions designed to reward specific behaviors: they were generating those behaviors. The institution's financial health was served. The patients were the mechanism by which that service was performed.

Ezekiel was not describing physicians when he wrote the words that open this chapter. He was describing shepherds who allowed themselves to rule with force and harshness rather than to tend the flock they had been given. The line between failing to tend and actively harming is a line this chapter does not need to locate precisely. What it has documented is that the flock entered the care of an institution that, by every measurable financial incentive, was structured to do something other than tend it.

IX. THE SCRIPTURE, PLACED AT THE CLOSE

Ezekiel 34 is not a comfort text. It is an indictment delivered by a prophet to the people responsible for the care of the vulnerable — and its verdict is that the failure of shepherds is not a lesser sin than active predation. The shepherd who does not strengthen the weak, who does not heal the sick, who does not seek the lost — who rules instead with force and harshness — stands under the same prophetic condemnation as the one who actively destroys.

The chapter that opened this book's Part Four documented the mechanism by which the global response to COVID-19 was organized. This chapter has documented what that organized response looked like from the inside of an American hospital — the financial signals, the protocol mandates, the treatment suppressions, the removal of advocates, and the institutional inertia that kept it all in place while the evidence against it accumulated in peer-reviewed journals that no one was permitted to act on within the institutional framework.

The reader who has followed this book from Chapter 1 does not need to be told what Ezekiel is describing. They have been reading it for twelve chapters.

The reader who has followed this book from the Introduction already knows where the rope leads and whose hand is holding it. Part Five documents what it looks like to take hold of it — the practical content of coming out, and the person who makes coming out more than a political act.

PRIMARY SOURCES FOR THIS CHAPTER

CARES Act and CMS Payment Incentives:

- Coronavirus Aid, Relief, and Economic Security Act (CARES Act), Pub. L. 116-136 (2020), Section 3710: "Medicare hospital inpatient prospective payment system add-on payment for COVID-19 patients during emergency period." Full text at congress.gov/116/plaws/publ136/PLAW-116publ136.pdf. Section 3710 is the specific provision establishing the 20 percent add-on.

- Centers for Medicare and Medicaid Services, "Additional Hospital

Payments for COVID-19 Patients," cms.gov. CMS documentation of the payment provisions implemented under Section 3710, including guidance on diagnosis coding and the add-on calculation.

- U.S. Senate Finance Committee Staff Report, "Follow the Money: COVID-19 Inpatient Hospital Payment Incentives," May 2022. Staff analysis raising questions about whether the CARES Act 20 percent add-on created perverse coding incentives. Available through senate.gov.

- Senator Scott Jensen's public statements and interviews, 2020, documented in Minnesota Star Tribune and Fox News reporting. Jensen is both a Minnesota state senator and a licensed physician; his statements about coding guidance from the Minnesota Department of Health were made in multiple public forums and are in the public record.

Ventilator Outcomes:

- Richardson, Safiya et al., "Presenting Characteristics, Comorbidities, and Outcomes Among 5700 Patients Hospitalized With COVID-19 in the New York City Area," *JAMA* 323(20), May 26, 2020. The Northwell Health system study documenting 88.1 percent mortality in ventilated COVID patients. Available at jamanetwork.com.

- Grasselli, Giacomo et al., "Baseline Characteristics and Outcomes of 1591 Patients Infected With SARS-CoV-2 Admitted to ICUs of the Lombardy Region, Italy," *JAMA* 323(16), April 2020. Italian ICU outcome data consistent with New York findings.

- Auld, Sara C. et al., "ICU and Ventilator Mortality Among Critically Ill Adults With Coronavirus Disease 2019," *Critical Care Medicine*, September 2020. Systematic analysis of ventilator mortality outcomes in the United States.

- Kyle-Sidell, Cameron, video statement published March 30,

2020, Maimonides Medical Center emergency physician. Available in archived form through multiple medical news outlets. Kyle-Sidell subsequently published in peer-reviewed forums describing the atypical respiratory presentation of COVID patients.

Remdesivir:

- U.S. Food and Drug Administration, "Emergency Use Authorization for Remdesivir," May 1, 2020. FDA.gov. The primary authorization document, available in full at fda.gov/media/137564/download.

- WHO Solidarity Trial Consortium, "Repurposed Antiviral Drugs for COVID-19 — Interim WHO Solidarity Trial Results," *New England Journal of Medicine* 383(24), October 8, 2020. The WHO's own trial results showing no statistically significant mortality benefit for remdesivir. Available at nejm.org.

- U.S. Food and Drug Administration, "FDA Approves First Treatment for COVID-19," October 22, 2020. FDA press release granting full approval to remdesivir — issued 14 days after publication of the Solidarity Trial results. Available at fda.gov.

- World Health Organization, "WHO Guidelines for COVID-19" updated November 2020 recommending against remdesivir in hospitalized patients, available at who.int.

- European Medicines Agency, "EMA review of remdesivir (Veklury) confirms findings of insufficient evidence for clinical benefit," April 2021. EMA statement documenting the agency's conclusion that evidence of mortality benefit remained inconclusive. Available at ema.europa.eu.

- Institute for Clinical and Economic Review, "Remdesivir for the Treatment of COVID-19: Effectiveness and Value," Final Evidence Report, May 2020. Cost-effectiveness analysis estimating production costs at $9-$91 per course. Available at icer.org.

Early Treatment Suppression:

- Senate Homeland Security Committee, Hearing on "Early Outpatient Treatment: An Essential Part of a COVID-19 Solution," December 8, 2020. Full hearing transcript and Dr. Pierre Kory's testimony are in the congressional record and available at hsgac.senate.gov.

- FDA guidance, "Why You Should Not Use Ivermectin to Treat or Prevent COVID-19," August 2021. Available at fda.gov. This is the FDA's own guidance document, including the "you are not a horse" framing.

- National Institutes of Health, "COVID-19 Treatment Guidelines: Ivermectin," last updated 2021. NIH guidelines panel's "neither for nor against" classification available at covid19treatmentguidelines.nih.gov.

- Kory, Pierre et al., "Review of the Emerging Evidence Demonstrating the Efficacy of Ivermectin in the Prophylaxis and Treatment of COVID-19," *American Journal of Therapeutics* 28(3), May/June 2021. Peer-reviewed publication of the evidence base Kory presented to the Senate. Available at ncbi.nlm.nih.gov.

Visitor Restriction Policies:

- Centers for Medicare and Medicaid Services, "CMS Guidance on COVID-19 Focused Infection Control Survey for Nursing Homes," June 2020. Non-binding CMS guidance on visitation. Available at cms.gov.

- Kunin, Marina, Bridget M. Engelhardt, and Thomas V. Perneger, "The Ethics of Visitor Restrictions During COVID-19," *New England Journal of Medicine*, June 18, 2020. Peer-reviewed perspective article on the humanitarian harm of blanket visitor restrictions.

- National Academy for State Health Policy, "COVID-19: Hospital

Visitor Restrictions by State," 2020-2021. State-by-state tracking of hospital visitor restriction policies during the pandemic. Available at nashp.org.

Comparative Mortality and Outcomes:

- Woolf, Steven H. et al., "Excess Deaths From COVID-19 and Other Causes, March-July 2020," *JAMA* 324(15), October 2020. Peer-reviewed analysis of excess mortality in the United States compared to expected all-cause mortality.

- Agrawal, Urvish K. et al., "Comparison of Mortality Outcomes After Early Treatment With Hydroxychloroquine Plus Azithromycin vs. Usual Care," *International Journal of Infectious Diseases*, 2021. Representative study from international early treatment literature.

- Lown Institute, analysis on COVID-19 outcomes and early treatment, published 2021. Available at lowninstitute.org.

- CDC WONDER database — CDC Wide-ranging Online Data for Epidemiologic Research. Excess death statistics, cause-of-death data, and state-level COVID mortality data. Available at wonder.cdc.gov.

Congressional Record:

- U.S. Senate Committee on Homeland Security and Governmental Affairs, "Early Outpatient Treatment of COVID-19" hearings, 2020-2021. Multiple hearing transcripts available at hsgac.senate.gov.

- Dr. Martin Makary's congressional testimonies, documented in House and Senate hearing records. Makary, a Johns Hopkins surgeon, testified on multiple occasions on early treatment and the institutional barriers to its study.

As with every chapter in this book, the reader who wants to verify these claims is directed to the primary documents, not to this author's summary of them. Every claim in this chapter traces to a government record, a peer-reviewed publication, a congressional transcript, or the published statements of the principals. The reader is invited to do what this book has asked from the first page: do not take this on faith. Look.

Chapter 13: The Pandemic Episode

DARPA, Gain-of-Function, the Lancet Letter, and the Congressional Record

"Be sure your sin will find you out."

— Numbers 32:23

The two chapters that precede this one documented the apparatus in operation: the global coordination mechanism that moved 190 countries in lockstep within days of a single declaration from Geneva, and the financial architecture inside American hospitals that converted the healing institution into an instrument of the response framework. Those chapters documented what the apparatus did.

This chapter documents where the apparatus came from.

Not in the sense of the century-long lineage that Part One through Three established — that lineage is complete. In the sense of the specific episode: the specific platform technology deployed on a global population, the specific research that preceded the outbreak, the specific management of the scientific record when questions about that research arose, and the specific mechanism by which people with a financial interest in a particular answer organized scientific consensus to produce that answer — while communicating through private channels specifically designed to leave no documentary trace.

The trace was found anyway.

Everything in this chapter is in the primary source record: congressional testimony under oath, FOIA-released documents obtained through litigation, federal audit findings, peer-reviewed scientific literature, and the published statements of the principals themselves. The reader who wants to verify any claim in this chapter is directed to those sources. This book does not require trust. It requires only the willingness to look.

I. THE PLATFORM: WHAT WAS BUILT AND WHO BUILT IT

To understand what was deployed in 2020, begin not in December 2019 but in 2011.

In that year, the Defense Advanced Research Projects Agency — DARPA, the research arm of the U.S. Department of Defense — launched a program called ADEPT: Autonomous Diagnostics to Enable Prevention and Therapeutics. The program's stated objective, in DARPA's own documentation, was to develop technologies to "rapidly identify and respond to threats posed by natural and engineered diseases and toxins," including "novel methods for rapidly manufacturing new types of vaccines."

The word *engineered* is in DARPA's own program description, as published on DARPA's own website.

In 2013, through the ADEPT program, DARPA awarded Moderna — then a small biotechnology startup with no approved products and no commercial revenue — $25 million to develop its messenger RNA platform. This award is documented in DARPA's public records, in Moderna's own SEC filings, in the published scientific literature, and in a Congressional Research Service report titled "mRNA Technologies: A Primer," available through the Library of Congress at congress.gov. It is not disputed by anyone. It is the foundational fact on which everything that follows depends: Moderna's mRNA technology was built, from its earliest stage, on defense research funding, for defense research purposes.

In 2016, DARPA initiated a successor program called the Pandemic Prevention Platform — P3 — as a direct extension of ADEPT.

DARPA's own program announcement describes P3 as aimed at developing the ADEPT work "into an entire system capable of halting the spread of any viral disease outbreak before it can escalate to pandemic status," with influenza, Zika, and Middle East Respiratory Syndrome as test cases. The stated goal was a deployable platform capable of producing effective countermeasures within sixty days of any novel viral threat.

By 2020, DARPA had invested approximately $400 million through ADEPT and P3 in nucleic acid vaccine technology.

A peer-reviewed retrospective cohort study published in the *British Medical Journal* in 2022 — drawing on federal grant databases and SEC filings — calculated the full public investment in mRNA Covid vaccine development. Of $337 million in pre-pandemic foundational research, 35 percent came from the NIH, 44 percent from BARDA, and 21 percent from the Department of Defense — which is DARPA. Three NIH scientists were listed as co-inventors on the foundational Moderna vaccine patent, which is documented in the patent's own filing record. The *BMJ* authors noted that NIH's "partnership and direct involvement in developing the covid-19 vaccine marketed by Moderna was so substantial" as to warrant co-inventorship status.

The platform technology deployed globally beginning in late 2020 was not a private-sector innovation brought to market through ordinary pharmaceutical development. It was a defense research program, funded by the Pentagon, built for the purpose of rapid mass deployment in response to biological threats — including, in DARPA's own published language, engineered ones — commercialized through an emergency regulatory framework and administered to billions of people.

The reader who has followed this book from Chapter 3 — which documented Operation Paperclip's transfer of the experimental ideology from Nazi Germany to American institutional soil — will recognize the institutional pathway. The specific technology is new. The movement of defense-funded biological research into civilian deployment through emergency frameworks, without the long-term safety data that ordinary approvals require, is not new. It is the pattern.

II. THE RESEARCH IN WUHAN: WHAT THE GRANTS FUNDED

Simultaneously with DARPA's mRNA program, a parallel funding stream was flowing through the National Institutes of Health to research on bat coronaviruses at the Wuhan Institute of Virology in China.

The mechanism was a New York-based nonprofit called EcoHealth Alliance, led by British zoologist Dr. Peter Daszak. Beginning in 2014, NIH awarded EcoHealth Alliance a grant — ultimately totaling approximately $3.7 million across multiple years — to study bat coronaviruses under a program titled "Understanding the Risk of Bat Coronavirus Emergence." Of this funding, approximately $600,000 to $750,000 was passed through as subawards to the Wuhan Institute of Virology. The grant was renewed for a five-year period in 2019.

This is documented in NIH's own grant records, in congressional testimony, and in 900 pages of grant proposals and progress reports obtained through FOIA litigation by *The Intercept*, published in September 2021.

What those documents revealed about the research was specific. Scientists working under the NIH grant combined genetic material from a parent coronavirus known as WIV1 with other viruses, creating chimeric hybrids. When tested in genetically engineered mice, three of the altered bat coronaviruses reproduced at rates far exceeding the original virus. In one experiment, the enhanced growth reached a factor of approximately 10,000 — four orders of magnitude, four log — above the rate of the original. The grant terms required EcoHealth to immediately report to NIH any unexpected viral growth exceeding one log. There is no record of this reporting occurring when the experiments produced the four-log result.

On October 20, 2021, Dr. Lawrence Tabak — principal deputy director of the NIH, the number-two official of the agency — sent a letter to Congress acknowledging that the NIH had funded gain-of-function research at the Wuhan Institute of Virology through its grant to EcoHealth Alliance.

This directly contradicted testimony given by Dr. Anthony Fauci to the United States Senate on May 11, 2021, in which he stated: "The NIH has not ever and does not now fund gain-of-function research in the Wuhan Institute of Virology."

Both statements are in the congressional record. They cannot both be true. Tabak subsequently testified under oath before the House Select Subcommittee on the Coronavirus Pandemic, reaffirming his admission. The Select Subcommittee reviewed more than one million pages of documents and interviewed more than a dozen witnesses over the course of its investigation.

On the same day — October 20, 2021 — that Tabak sent his letter to Congress acknowledging the gain-of-function research, the NIH removed its longstanding public definition of gain-of-function from its website. The definition that was removed had read: "a type of research that modifies a biological agent so that it confers new or enhanced activity to that agent." The Select Subcommittee documented the timing of this removal in its published report. The NIH has not explained the coincidence.

EcoHealth Alliance's Year 5 progress report — the report that contained the data about the chimeric coronavirus experiments producing the four-log growth result — was due to NIH on September 30, 2019. The report was not submitted until August 3, 2021: nearly two years late. The Select Subcommittee documented this delay in its May 2024 interim report. The report was submitted only after congressional pressure made non-submission untenable.

The HHS Office of Inspector General conducted an eighteen-month audit of EcoHealth Alliance grants from 2014 to 2021, totaling $8 million. The OIG found that NIH "did not effectively monitor or take timely action to address" compliance problems with EcoHealth's grants. The OIG recommended that the Wuhan Institute of Virology be debarred from future NIH funding.

In May 2024, the House Select Subcommittee recommended that EcoHealth Alliance president Dr. Peter Daszak be debarred from federal funding and criminally investigated. The Department of Health and Human Services subsequently suspended EcoHealth's funding and initiated debarment proceedings. Daszak was banned from receiving federal funding for five years.

III. THE SUPPRESSION: HOW THE NARRATIVE WAS ORGANIZED

On February 19, 2020 — six weeks into public awareness of the outbreak — a letter signed by 27 scientists was published in *The Lancet*, one of the most prestigious medical journals in the world. The letter expressed "solidarity with all scientists and health professionals in China" and stated that the signatories "strongly condemn conspiracy theories suggesting that COVID-19 does not have a natural origin." Three signatories of the letter were EcoHealth Alliance employees, a conflict not disclosed in the letter itself.

The letter had an immediate and decisive effect. *Vanity Fair* journalist Katherine Eban, reporting in June 2021 from primary documents, wrote that it had a "chilling effect" on the scientific community by framing anyone who raised the lab-leak question as conducting the work of conspiracy theorists. Scientists who had intended to investigate the question described pulling back after the letter appeared.

The letter was organized by Dr. Peter Daszak — the head of EcoHealth Alliance, whose organization had funded the gain-of-function research at the Wuhan Institute of Virology, and who had a direct financial and institutional interest in the outcome of the origins question. He did not disclose this conflict of interest in the letter.

When *The Lancet* subsequently invited the signatories to re-evaluate their competing interests, Daszak disclosed in an email — obtained through FOIA and later made public — that he had composed the letter after his "collaborators" in China asked for a "show of support." Documents released by *The Intercept* showed that Daszak had specifically advised Dr. Ralph Baric, a prominent gain-of-function researcher and EcoHealth collaborator, against signing: "because we need to put it out in a way that doesn't link it back to our collaboration so we maximize an independent voice."

The goal, in Daszak's own words, was to create the appearance of independent scientific consensus while deliberately concealing the signatories' financial and institutional relationships to the research under scrutiny.

The Lancet itself noted in an addendum that Daszak "should certainly have declared his competing interests right at the beginning."

Three of the original letter's signatories subsequently reversed their positions publicly. Peter Palese of the Icahn School of Medicine stated he believed "a thorough investigation about the origin of the COVID-19 virus is needed." Charles Calisher told ABC News he had "completely changed his position." Bernard Roizman stated: "I'm convinced that what happened is that the virus was brought to a lab, they started to work with it...and some sloppy individual brought it out."

IV. THE PROXIMAL ORIGIN: WHAT THE AUTHORS SAID IN PRIVATE

Parallel to the *Lancet* letter, a second paper was published in *Nature Medicine* in March 2020, titled "The Proximal Origin of SARS-CoV-2." This paper became the dominant scientific citation used by government officials and media organizations to dismiss the lab-leak hypothesis as conspiracy. It was accessed online more than 5.7 million times and cited by more than 2,000 outlets.

Unredacted emails obtained through FOIA litigation by *The Intercept*, released after more than a year of litigation, revealed what was happening privately among the paper's authors in the weeks before they wrote it.

In late January 2020 — before the paper existed — Dr. Kristian Andersen of Scripps Research wrote to Dr. Anthony Fauci and NIH Director Francis Collins that when examining the virus "really closely," "some of the features (potentially) look engineered" and that he and colleagues "all find the genome inconsistent with expectations from evolutionary theory." Dr. Robert Garry, another of the paper's eventual authors, wrote that the furin cleavage site — a specific genetic feature of SARS-CoV-2 with no close analog in any known natural coronavirus relative — "bothers me."

These private communications were written on January 31 and February 1, 2020.

On February 1, a conference call was convened between Fauci,

Collins, Andersen, Garry, and the other virologists who would write the "Proximal Origin" paper. The substance of this call was heavily redacted in initial FOIA releases. The unredacted version — made available only after sustained congressional pressure — confirmed, in Fauci's own subsequent congressional testimony, that it was "a very productive back-and-forth conversation where some on the call felt it could possibly be an engineered virus."

By March 17, 2020 — six weeks after privately expressing that the virus looked potentially engineered — Andersen, Garry, and their colleagues published "The Proximal Origin of SARS-CoV-2" publicly characterizing the lab-leak hypothesis as not credible. The paper's final acknowledgments thanked Fauci and Collins for their "advice and leadership."

The sequence is now in the unredacted documentary record: scientists privately expressing that the virus looked engineered → conference call with the NIH's two most senior officials → paper publicly dismissing those exact concerns.

This is not inference. It is in the emails, which are FOIA-released documents in the public domain.

V. THE PRIVATE CHANNELS: MAKING EMAILS DISAPPEAR

The management of the origins narrative did not stop at published letters and papers.

Dr. David Morens was the Senior Advisor to Dr. Fauci at the National Institute of Allergy and Infectious Diseases — the number-two official in Fauci's office. Emails obtained by the House Select Subcommittee documented Morens in regular communication with Peter Daszak through what Morens described as a "secret back channel." The emails revealed a pattern of behavior that the Select Subcommittee described as "overwhelming evidence" of "serious misconduct and potentially illegal actions."

In one email, Morens wrote to Daszak: "I can either send stuff to Tony on his private gmail, or hand it to him at work or at his house. He is too smart to let colleagues send him stuff that could cause trouble."

In another, Morens wrote that he "always try[ies] to communicate over gmail because my NIH email is FOIA'd constantly."

In another, he described that he knew "how to make emails disappear after I am FOIA'd."

In another, addressing the origins question directly: "Tony doesn't want his fingerprints on origin stories."

These statements are in emails. The emails are in the congressional record. The House Select Subcommittee concluded that Morens had "engaged in serious misconduct and potentially illegal actions" including "undermining the operations of the U.S. government, unlawfully deleting federal COVID-19 records, using a personal email to avoid the Freedom of Information Act."

The reader who remembers Chapter 4 of this book — in which CIA Director Richard Helms ordered the destruction of approximately 20,000 documents related to the MKUltra program before the Church Committee could subpoena them — will recognize the operating principle. The specific technology for record destruction changes. The institutional impulse to destroy the record when accountability approaches does not.

Be sure your sin will find you out.

The Morens emails were found. The EcoHealth progress report — submitted nearly two years late — was found. The unredacted February 1 conference call record was found. The FOIA emails in which Daszak described concealing the letter's authorship to "maximize an independent voice" were found. The gap between what Fauci told the Senate and what Tabak subsequently testified under oath is in the congressional record.

The verse that opens this chapter is from the book of Numbers. Moses is addressing two and a half tribes of Israel who want to settle east of the Jordan River rather than cross into the promised land. His warning to them is not theological abstraction. It is a statement about the nature of hidden things: they do not remain hidden. The record accumulates. The documents surface. The subordinates, under oath, contradict the official story.

It has always worked this way. It worked this way here.

VI. THE INTELLIGENCE COMMUNITY'S ASSESSMENT

By 2023, three U.S. government agencies had formally assessed that Covid-19 most likely originated from a laboratory incident.

The **Federal Bureau of Investigation assessed with* moderate confidence* that the pandemic resulted from a potential laboratory incident in Wuhan. FBI Director Christopher Wray confirmed this publicly in a February 28, 2023 interview.

The **Department of Energy assessed with* low confidence* that Covid-19 likely originated from a laboratory leak. The DOE oversees the national laboratory network and has substantial internal expertise in biological sciences and research biosafety.

The **Central Intelligence Agency** subsequently revised its internal assessment to lean toward a laboratory origin, based on reinterpretation of existing evidence.

The U.S. intelligence community remained divided: four other agencies assessed with low confidence that the virus likely emerged naturally, and one was unable to reach a conclusion. No agency claimed high confidence in either direction. The division is itself meaningful: the unanimous confidence that characterized the official public dismissal of the lab-leak hypothesis in 2020 — branded a conspiracy theory by institutional voices citing the *Lancet* letter and the *Nature Medicine* paper — was not the intelligence community's actual assessment.

The Senate Health, Education, Labor and Pensions Committee's minority staff investigation, reviewing hundreds of publicly available scientific studies and interviewing dozens of subject matter experts, concluded in its 2022–2023 interim reports that "it appears reasonable to conclude that the COVID-19 pandemic was, more likely than not, the result of a research-related incident." The investigation noted that no naturally occurring virus with the same genetic composition as SARS-CoV-2 has ever been found in nature; that epidemiological evidence suggests the virus was circulating in Wuhan before the first known cases connected to the Huanan wet market; and that Chinese authorities have persistently refused to cooperate with independent investigation.

Former CDC Director Robert Redfield — himself a virologist with decades of biosafety experience — testified before Congress: "Based on my initial analysis of the data, I came to believe and I still believe today that it indicates that Covid-19 more likely was a result of an accidental lab leak than the result of a natural spillover event. This conclusion is based primarily on the biology of the virus itself."

Dr. Robert Garry — one of the "Proximal Origin" authors who had publicly dismissed the lab-leak hypothesis — testified before the Senate: "I really can't think of a plausible natural scenario when you get from the bat virus, or one very similar to it, COVID-19, where you insert exactly four amino acids, 12 nucleotides, and all have to be added at the exact same time to gain this function. I just can't figure out how this gets accomplished in nature." He added:

"It's not crackpot to suggest this could have happened, given the gain of function research we know was happening in Wuhan."

This is the same Robert Garry who, on February 1, 2020, wrote privately that the furin cleavage site "bothers me" — and who, six weeks later, co-authored the paper that became the primary institutional citation for dismissing the lab-leak hypothesis.

VII. THE DEPLOYMENT: EMERGENCY AUTHORIZATION AND WHAT IT BYPASSED

Whatever the origin of SARS-CoV-2, the response it triggered deployed the mRNA platform — built on a decade of defense research funding, never before approved for widespread human use — through a regulatory pathway that explicitly set aside the long-term safety requirements that govern ordinary pharmaceutical approvals.

The Emergency Use Authorization framework, established under the Public Health Service Act, allows the FDA to authorize medical countermeasures before full approval when a public health emergency has been declared, there is no adequate alternative, and potential benefits outweigh potential risks. The framework exists because genuine emergencies sometimes demand action before complete evidence is in hand. It is not inherently improper.

What it does not require — and what was not provided for the mRNA Covid vaccines — is the multi-year follow-up safety data that forms the backbone of standard pharmaceutical approval. The full regulatory review process for a novel vaccine platform takes between ten and fifteen years. The mRNA Covid vaccines moved from the beginning of human clinical trials to mass global deployment in approximately twelve months.

The Congressional Research Service's mRNA Technologies primer documents that DARPA's decade of investment in the platform was what made this speed structurally possible. The platform was not created in response to Covid. It was created in defense research infrastructure between 2011 and 2020, under programs explicitly designed for rapid mass deployment, repurposed when the pandemic arrived.

The total U.S. public investment in mRNA Covid vaccines — from foundational research through vaccine supply procurement — was documented at $31.9 billion in the *BMJ* retrospective study. Moderna received $10.8 billion in U.S. government funding. Pfizer's partner BioNTech received $445 million in German government funding; the U.S. government purchased $20.4 billion in Pfizer-BioNTech vaccine supply.

DARPA investigated Moderna in 2020 for allegedly failing to disclose its DARPA funding in patent applications — a legal requirement under the Bayh-Dole Act, which governs inventions developed with federal funding. The pharmaceutical watchdog organization Knowledge Ecology International documented that none of 126 patents granted to Moderna referenced the initial DARPA funding, despite published academic papers and Moderna's own SEC disclosures from the same period acknowledging the grants. This is documented in KEI's letter to DARPA and the Secretary of Defense, cited in *Health Policy Watch*'s reporting.

The pattern is what it has always been in every chapter of this book: public funding builds the foundational technology, private companies hold the patents and collect the revenue, the public assumes the risk. The institutional pathway from Rockefeller's capture of American medical education to DARPA's creation of the mRNA platform runs in a straight line. The beneficiaries change. The structure does not.

VIII. WHAT THE RECORD ESTABLISHES AND WHAT IT DOES NOT

The evidentiary discipline that has governed this book from Chapter 1 requires this distinction to be made plainly.

The primary source record establishes:

The mRNA vaccine platform deployed globally in 2020 was built on DARPA defense research funding, confirmed in DARPA's own public records, federal grant databases, a Congressional Research Service report, and peer-reviewed scientific literature. Three NIH researchers were co-inventors on Moderna's foundational patent.

NIH funded gain-of-function research on bat coronaviruses at the Wuhan Institute of Virology through EcoHealth Alliance — confirmed in the sworn testimony of former NIH principal deputy director Lawrence Tabak before Congress, in the HHS Office of Inspector General's audit, and in the House Select Subcommittee's published findings.

Dr. Fauci testified to the Senate in May 2021 that NIH had never funded gain-of-function research at the WIV. Dr. Tabak testified under oath that it had. Both statements are in the congressional record.

NIH removed its definition of gain-of-function from its website on the same day Tabak reported EcoHealth's experiments to Congress — confirmed in the Select Subcommittee's published report.

Dr. Peter Daszak organized the *Lancet* letter branding the lab-leak hypothesis a "conspiracy theory" while concealing his organization's financial relationship to the Wuhan research, and did so at the request of Chinese collaborators seeking a "show of support" — confirmed in FOIA-released emails.

The "Proximal Origin" authors who publicly dismissed the lab-leak hypothesis had privately expressed to Fauci and Collins that the virus looked potentially engineered, days before writing the paper — confirmed in unredacted emails obtained through FOIA litigation by *The Intercept*.

Dr. David Morens, Senior Advisor to Fauci, used personal email to avoid FOIA, communicated with Daszak through a private "secret back channel," and documented instructions for making emails disappear after FOIA requests — confirmed in emails obtained by the House Select Subcommittee.

The FBI, the Department of Energy, and the CIA have each assessed that Covid-19 most likely originated from a laboratory incident — confirmed in public statements by FBI Director Christopher Wray and in intelligence community assessments.

The primary source record does not establish:

That SARS-CoV-2 was intentionally engineered as a weapon. The FBI and DOE assessments indicate a likely laboratory accident — an accidental release — not a deliberate act. The specific viruses documented in EcoHealth's funded research are genetically too distant from SARS-CoV-2 to be its direct progenitor, based on the published genetic record. The origin question has not been definitively resolved.

This book will not claim what the evidence does not support. What the evidence does support is sufficient.

IX. THE CONVERGENCE: WHAT THE LINEAGE REQUIRES US TO SEE

Read the documented record of the Covid episode in isolation and it looks like the convergence of recognizable institutional failures: inadequate oversight of a risky research grant, a conflict of interest disclosure failure in a scientific journal, an NIH official using personal email to avoid records requests, intelligence agencies reaching different conclusions from the same evidence under political pressure.

These things happen. They are individually explicable.

Read the same documented record against the lineage established in the preceding twelve chapters, and the pattern comes into focus with a specificity that individual explanations cannot account for.

The deployment of experimental biological technology on a non-consenting population through an emergency regulatory framework that bypasses standard long-term safety requirements — that is the exact pattern documented in Chapter 3 through Chapter 5. The mechanism has changed from plutonium injections to mRNA. The assumption has not changed: that under sufficiently urgent circumstances, the requirement for informed consent and long-term safety evaluation can be set aside. The Nuremberg Code that was adopted in 1947 specifically in response to the Nazi medical experiments said voluntary consent "is absolutely essential." The EUA framework says potential benefits must outweigh potential risks — a substantially different standard, applied to a novel platform technology deployed to billions.

The organization of scientific consensus to suppress inquiry into institutional culpability — Daszak convening the *Lancet* letter while concealing his conflict, the *Nature Medicine* authors privately expressing concern about engineered features and then publicly dismissing those concerns — is the exact pattern documented in Chapter 6's suppression architecture. The specific technique varies by era. The function is identical.

Federal officials communicating through private channels to avoid FOIA, deleting records, managing public narrative to protect institutional interests while a program under their authority caused harm — that is the pattern from the CIA's destruction of the

MKUltra records in 1973 to David Morens instructing colleagues on making emails disappear in 2021. The Church Committee found it. The House Select Subcommittee found it again, in the same federal bureaucracy, nearly fifty years later.

The mRNA platform built in DARPA defense research infrastructure and deployed commercially through emergency authorization is the institutional pathway that the entire lineage of this book has traced: classified or defense-funded research migrating to civilian deployment without the accountability structures that govern ordinary pharmaceutical development. Chapter 3 documented Operation Paperclip's transfer of the experimental ideology from Nazi Germany to American soil. Chapter 13 documents the transfer of a decade of Pentagon biological research to global mass deployment in twelve months.

Each element of the Covid episode, taken alone, can be explained by the ordinary mechanisms of institutional failure, regulatory capture, and scientific careerism. The grant that wasn't monitored. The journal letter whose author didn't disclose his conflict. The official who used personal email to avoid FOIA. These things happen in bureaucracies. They have individual explanations.

What does not have an individual explanation is the convergence. The concentration of every element of the documented seventy-year lineage — operating simultaneously, on the human biological template, at global scale, at precisely the moment when the platform technology for doing so became available — is not adequately explained by the sum of its individual parts.

The Introduction to this book named what explains it. John 10:10 named it first. The thief comes only to steal and kill and destroy. The men and women documented across thirteen chapters did not originate what they served. They sold themselves to it — for wealth, for protection, for the intoxicating certainty of being on the winning side. The documentary record does not establish their conscious awareness of what they served. It establishes the consistency of what they produced. And what they produced, across a hundred years and a hundred institutions, is a single coherent assault on human biological sovereignty, human cognitive freedom, and human life.

The documents are in front of you. The lineage is complete. The reader who has followed from the Introduction already knows what the convergence means. What remains is the question the evidence demands of every person who sees it clearly: not what it is, but what you will do now that you know.

X. THE CLOSE OF PART FOUR

Part Four is now complete.

Chapter 11 documented the mechanism by which the global response was coordinated — WHO, IHR, GAVI, CEPI, the Gates Foundation, the WEF — and the exercise, six weeks before the first Covid cases, at which that coordination was rehearsed.

Chapter 12 documented what that coordinated response looked like inside an American hospital — the financial incentives, the protocol mandates, the suppression of early treatment, the removal of family advocates at the moment of maximum patient vulnerability.

Chapter 13 has documented where the apparatus itself came from — the defense-funded platform technology, the NIH-funded research in Wuhan, the organized suppression of the origins question, and the private channels specifically designed to ensure that when accountability came, the documentary record would not be there to meet it.

The record was there anyway. The record is always there. That is the meaning of the verse that opens this chapter, and it applies not only to Peter Daszak's emails or David Morens's instructions on making documents disappear. It applies to everything in this book. The apparatus was built in the open, documented in the open, and is available for anyone willing to look. The suppression has never been total. The witnesses have never been fully silenced. The record has always been recoverable.

The reader who has followed from the Introduction has now seen the full case. The ideology built in Chapter 1. The medical monopoly constructed in Chapter 2. The experimental methodology transferred in Chapter 3. The programs proven on American citizens in Chapters 4 and 5. The suppression architecture refined in Chapter 6. The regulatory agencies captured in Chapter 7. The food system locked down in Chapter 8. The childhood health infrastructure converted in Chapter 9. The enforcement network documented in Chapter 10. The global coordination mechanism deployed in Chapter 11. The healing institution converted into an instrument in Chapter 12. And now, in Chapter 13: the specific episode in which all of it ran at once, at global scale, and the record of what was done to conceal it accumulating in FOIA requests and congressional testimony faster than it could be destroyed.

This is what the book set out to document. It has documented it.

The Introduction named the thief. The Introduction named the rope. The reader who arrived at Chapter 1 knowing those names has spent thirteen chapters watching the evidence confirm them. The reader who arrived skeptical has spent thirteen chapters following the documentation to wherever it leads. Both readers arrive at Part Five in the same place: in possession of the full evidentiary record, and faced with the question that record demands.

Not: what is behind this? The Introduction answered that.

Not: is the rope real? The Introduction named it.

The question Part Five addresses is the one that remains after those are answered: what do you do now?

That is a different kind of question. It is not answered by documentation. It is answered by decision. And Part Five — the exit, and the one who makes the exit possible — is where the decision lives.

PRIMARY SOURCES FOR THIS CHAPTER

Congressional Records and Government Reports:

- House Select Subcommittee on the Coronavirus Pandemic, *An Evaluation of the Evidence Surrounding EcoHealth Alliance, Inc.'s Research Activities*, Interim Staff Report, May 2024. Available: oversight.house.gov. The primary congressional investigation finding, after reviewing more than one million pages of documents, that NIH funded gain-of-function research at WIV and that EcoHealth's leadership engaged in misconduct.

- House Select Subcommittee on the Coronavirus Pandemic, Hearing: "Overseeing the Overseers: A Hearing with NIH Deputy Director Lawrence Tabak," May 2024. Tabak's sworn testimony acknowledging NIH funded gain-of-function research at WIV. Available: congress.gov.

- U.S. Senate Committee on Health, Education, Labor and Pensions, Minority Staff, *An Analysis of the Origins of COVID-19*, Interim Report, October 2022. The Senate investigation concluding that a research-related incident was more likely than not the pandemic's origin. Available: help.senate.gov.

- U.S. Department of Health and Human Services, Office of Inspector General, Audit of NIH Grants to EcoHealth Alliance, 2023. The federal audit finding that NIH "did not effectively monitor or take timely action to address" compliance problems with EcoHealth grants. Available: oig.hhs.gov.

- Lawrence Tabak letter to Congress, October 20, 2021. The NIH's written acknowledgment that EcoHealth Alliance experiments at WIV increased the replication of chimeric coronaviruses in humanized mice — published and widely reported October 21, 2021.

- Congressional Research Service, *mRNA Technologies: A Primer*, R47112. Available: congress.gov. Documents DARPA's 2013 $25 million award to Moderna and the full federal investment in mRNA platform development.

- FBI Director Christopher Wray, interview confirming FBI's "moderate confidence" assessment of laboratory origin, February 28, 2023. Transcript available through FBI.gov and reporting by *Fox News*.

- Former CDC Director Robert Redfield, congressional testimony, March 8, 2023, House Select Subcommittee on the Coronavirus Pandemic. Full transcript available: oversight.house.gov.

FOIA-Released Documents:

- NIH grant documents and EcoHealth Alliance progress reports, obtained through FOIA litigation by *The Intercept*, published September 2021. Includes EcoHealth Year 5 progress report submitted nearly two years late, containing data on chimeric coronavirus experiments. Available: theintercept.com.

- Unredacted NIH emails, obtained through FOIA litigation by *The Intercept*, published January 2023. Documents the January 31–February 1, 2020 communications between Andersen, Garry, Fauci, and Collins in which authors privately expressed that SARS-CoV-2 looked potentially engineered — days before they wrote the paper dismissing that possibility. Available: theintercept.com.

- Peter Daszak emails, obtained by the House Select Subcommittee, documenting the "secret back channel" with David Morens, Daszak's instruction to Baric not to sign the Lancet letter to preserve "an independent voice," and Morens's statements about communicating over Gmail to avoid FOIA and knowing "how to make emails disappear." Available: oversight.house.gov.

- Anthony Fauci emails, obtained by BuzzFeed News and *The Washington Post* through FOIA, published June 2021. Available: buzzfeednews.com.

Peer-Reviewed Scientific Literature:

- Galkina Cleary, E., et al., "US public investment in development of mRNA covid-19 vaccines: retrospective cohort study," *BMJ*, 2022. Documents the full scope of public funding in mRNA vaccine development, with 35% from NIH, 44% from BARDA, 21% from DOD. Documents three NIH researchers listed as co-inventors on Moderna's foundational patent. Available: bmj.com.

- Andersen, K.G., Rambaut, A., Lipkin, W.I., Holmes, E.C., Garry, R.F., "The proximal origin of SARS-CoV-2," *Nature Medicine* 26, March 2020. The paper itself, whose private genesis was documented in subsequently released FOIA emails. Available: nature.com.

Lancet Letter and Its Aftermath:

- Calisher, C. et al., "Statement in support of the scientists, public health professionals, and medical professionals of China combatting COVID-19," *The Lancet* 395, February 19, 2020. The original letter. Available: thelancet.com.

- *The Lancet* addendum noting Daszak "should certainly have declared his competing interests right at the beginning," published September 2021. Available: thelancet.com.

- Eban, Katherine, "The Lab-Leak Theory: Inside the Fight to Uncover COVID-19's Origins," *Vanity Fair*, June 2021. Based on primary document review, documenting the chilling effect of the Lancet letter and the internal conflict-of-interest suppression. Available: vanityfair.com.

DARPA Program Documentation:

- DARPA, Autonomous Diagnostics to Enable Prevention and Therapeutics (ADEPT) program documentation. Available: darpa.mil. Original program description including the reference to "engineered diseases and toxins."

- DARPA, Pandemic Prevention Platform (P3) program announcement, 2016. Available: darpa.mil.

EcoHealth Debarment and Federal Action:

- Department of Health and Human Services, Notice of Proposed Debarment of EcoHealth Alliance and Peter Daszak, 2023–2024. Documents the formal federal action taken following the OIG audit and Select Subcommittee investigation.

- Knowledge Ecology International, letter to DARPA and Secretary of Defense regarding Moderna's alleged failure to disclose federal funding in patent applications, 2020. Documents the Bayh-Dole compliance question. Available: keionline.org.

The reader is directed first to the primary documents, not to this author's account of them. Every claim in this chapter is supported by a government record, a congressional transcript, a FOIA-released document, or peer-reviewed scientific literature. The congressional record is permanent. The FOIA documents are public. The primary sources do not require trust in any author, including this one. They require only the willingness to read.

Chapter 14: The Exit

What Coming Out of the System Actually Looks Like

"Come out of her, my people, lest you take part in her sins, lest you share in her plagues."

— Revelation 18:4

The Introduction to this book planted this verse without context. The reader who encountered it there was curious or was not, recognized it or did not, and moved into the evidence either way.

The reader who arrives at this verse now has thirteen chapters of documentation behind it. The *her* the verse names has been described in institutional detail: the eugenics movement's foundation, the medical capture, the experimental programs, the suppression architecture, the regulatory revolving door, the food system, the childhood vaccine schedule, the Epstein enforcement network, the global coordination, the hospital protocols, the platform technology built for deployment and deployed. The command to come out is not abstract. The thing to come out of has a documented shape.

The command is also not easy. It has never been easy. Babylon's economic power, in the text Revelation 18 describes in the verses surrounding this one, is precisely its capacity to make departure feel impossible — because the wealth of nations flows through it, because its products are everywhere, because leaving means losing the comfort and security and status that participation provides. The text does not minimize this. It acknowledges it and commands departure anyway.

This chapter does the same. The exit is real. The exit is not comfortable. And the exit is not primarily a lifestyle choice — it is, as this book has argued from the first chapter, a decision about whose purposes you will serve with the body that was breathed into existence by the God who made it.

What follows is not a self-help program. It is the documented record of what the system suppressed, organized into the categories it suppressed hardest. The documented suppression is itself evidence. The system does not suppress what does not threaten it.

I. FOOD: WHAT THE SYSTEM SUPPRESSED AND WHAT REMAINS

Chapter 8 documented how the food system was captured — the purchased dietary science, the seed patents, the chemical agriculture built on suppressed safety data, the processed food engineered for addiction rather than nourishment. The capture was systematic. The alternatives it suppressed were equally systematic.

Seed sovereignty. The practice of seed saving — selecting the best plants from each harvest, storing their seeds, replanting them the following season — sustained every human civilization for ten thousand years before the patent system ended it for anyone using commercial varieties. It did not disappear. It was driven out of industrial agriculture and into an underground of seed libraries, seed swaps, and regional seed networks that has persisted and, in the past decade, grown.

The Organic Seed Alliance, the Seed Savers Exchange, and regional seed libraries maintained by agricultural extension programs and independent organizations have preserved tens of thousands of open-pollinated, non-patented seed varieties that are available to home gardeners and small farmers outside the corporate seed system. The Svalbard Global Seed Vault holds more than 1.4 million seed samples as a backup for this biological heritage. These are documented, operational, accessible resources. Growing food from open-pollinated seed is legal. Saving seed from open-pollinated varieties is legal. The corporate seed system's dominance is structural, not coercive — it operates through the managed dependency of the industrial farmer, not through the prohibition of alternatives.

The home garden is the minimum-scale exit. It is also, in the framework this book has documented, an act with a specific meaning: the person who grows food from open-pollinated seed, saves that seed, and replants it has exited the portion of the food system that patent law captured. That exit scales. Community gardens, CSA shares from farms that use open-pollinated seed, farmers' markets, and regional food networks all operate outside the corporate seed-and-chemical system at varying scales of accessibility.

Nutritional science outside the guidelines. Chapter 8 documented how the sugar industry purchased the dietary science that shaped the USDA's nutritional guidelines for sixty years, suppressing the fat-versus-sugar debate and producing the low-fat, high-carbohydrate dietary recommendations that contributed to the chronic disease epidemic the pharmaceutical system then managed. The suppressed science was not destroyed. It was documented in peer-reviewed journals that lacked the institutional backing to compete with the purchased consensus.

The JAMA Internal Medicine paper that documented the Sugar Research Foundation's funding of research designed to exonerate sugar — published in 2016 — established the mechanism of suppression in peer-reviewed form. The nutritional science that the guidelines suppressed is accessible. The work of researchers including Gary Taubes (*Good Calories, Bad Calories*, Anchor Books, 2008), Nina Teicholz (*The Big Fat Surprise*, Simon & Schuster, 2014), and the primary research literature they draw on documents the evidence base for dietary approaches — whole food, minimally processed, reduced refined carbohydrate — that the USDA guidelines have systematically underemphasized. These are not fringe sources. Taubes and Teicholz draw on peer-reviewed literature and have been published by major commercial publishers. Their work has been reviewed, criticized, and defended in the scientific literature.

The exit from the captured dietary guidelines is reading the science the guidelines suppressed. The primary literature is in the National Library of Medicine's PubMed database, freely searchable. The reader who wants to understand what the evidence actually shows about dietary fat, refined carbohydrates, and chronic disease has access to the same journals the Sugar Research Foundation paid to suppress the truth in. The suppression was never total. The record was always recoverable.

**The practical floor.* The minimum viable exit from the captured food system is: whole food, locally sourced where accessible, grown from non-patented seed where possible, processed as little as possible before consumption. This is not a novel insight. It is what every human being who was not pharmed ate for most of human history. The system spent a century making it feel complicated. It is not complicated. It was made to feel that way by the industry that profits from its replacement.

II. MEDICINE: WHAT OPERATES OUTSIDE THE PHARMACEUTICAL FRAMEWORK

Chapter 2 documented the Flexner restructuring's elimination of the competing traditions of American medicine. Chapter 7 documented the capture of the regulatory agencies. Chapter 12 documented the hospital protocols of 2020. The pharmaceutical framework is not the only framework available to the patient who chooses to look outside it.

Direct Primary Care. The direct primary care model — in which a patient pays a monthly membership fee directly to a physician, bypassing insurance billing entirely — has grown to more than 2,000 practices in the United States as of the most recent estimates, covering an estimated two to four million patients. The DPC Journal and the Direct Primary Care Alliance maintain directories of participating physicians. The model is documented in peer-reviewed health policy literature as producing significantly higher physician availability, longer appointment times, lower rates of specialist referral, and lower total healthcare costs for enrolled patients compared to standard fee-for-service insurance-based primary care.

The mechanism is important: a physician in a standard practice bills insurance companies for each service, creating volume incentives that reward brief appointments and high patient loads. A DPC physician bills a flat monthly membership fee — typically between $50 and $150 — and maintains a much smaller patient panel. The financial incentive is not volume. It is the patient's sustained health, because a patient who stays healthy requires less of the physician's time. The incentive structure is the inverse of the standard pharmaceutical model.

This is not a cure for the pharmaceutical capture. It is a partial exit from the incentive structure that the capture created. A DPC physician is still trained in pharmaceutical medicine and still operates within the pharmaceutical culture. But the financial separation from the insurance billing system removes one layer of the institutional pressure the captured model creates.

Informed consent as practice, not formality. Chapter 9 documented the childhood vaccine schedule's departure from the conditions of genuine informed consent. Chapter 12 documented the hospital protocols in which patients received treatments under conditions that made meaningful consent structurally unavailable.

Informed consent is documented in the medical ethics literature as a clinical practice — not a form to sign but an ongoing conversation in which the patient understands what is being proposed, what the alternatives are, what the evidence supports, and what the evidence does not support.

The patient who understands this has a different relationship to the institution. The right to a second opinion is legally recognized in every state. The right to refuse treatment — including treatment recommended under institutional protocol — is legally recognized. The right to access your own medical records is codified in federal law under HIPAA. The patient who exercises these rights is not a difficult patient. They are a patient practicing the minimum requirements of informed consent that the Nuremberg Code established in 1947.

The specific practical tools: maintaining your own complete medical history in a format you control, independent of any institution's electronic records system; understanding the difference between a recommended treatment and a mandated one; knowing that you have the right to ask any physician — including in an emergency room — what a proposed treatment is, what the alternatives are, and what the evidence shows. The patient who walks into a hospital with a family advocate, a personal medical record, and the knowledge of their rights is a fundamentally different patient from the one Chapter 12 documented entering the Covid-era hospital alone, uninformed, and isolated.

**The suppressed early treatment evidence.* Chapter 12 documented the suppression of early treatment options during the Covid period — not their clinical efficacy, which remains contested in the peer-reviewed literature, but the mechanism of suppression. The broader principle the suppression illustrated applies to the standard medical model throughout: the off-patent, inexpensive, nutritionally-based, or lifestyle-based intervention has no pharmaceutical champion funding the trials that would establish its evidence base. The absence of evidence for an approach whose proponents cannot afford to fund the trials is not the same as evidence of absence of effect.

The National Library of Medicine's PubMed database contains the primary research literature on nutritional approaches to chronic disease, on exercise and metabolic health, on sleep and immune function, on the relationship between gut microbiome diversity and chronic illness — research that the pharmaceutical model has no financial incentive to translate into clinical guidelines. This research is available, free, to any patient willing to read primary literature. A physician who practices evidence-based medicine is required to consider the evidence. The patient who brings that evidence to a clinical encounter is practicing the minimum standard of informed participation in their own care.

**The limits of the exit.* This chapter does not claim that the exit from the pharmaceutical framework is complete or that the alternatives it describes are adequate substitutes for the full range of medical care. Trauma surgery is not replaceable by any alternative tradition. Certain bacterial infections require antibiotics. The pharmaceutical model has produced genuine advances — selective, real, documented — that this book does not dispute. What the exit offers is not the replacement of medicine with its alternatives. It is the reclamation of the patient's role as the primary decision-maker in their own care, operating with full information about what the system's financial incentives are and what the evidence outside those incentives shows.

The patient who is pharmed is the patient who has been managed into chronic dependence on the system's products without understanding the alternatives. The patient who is not pharmed is the patient who knows the difference between what the evidence supports and what the system's incentives produce, and who makes decisions accordingly. The knowledge is available. The decision is the patient's.

III. COMMUNITY: THE DOCUMENTED RESILIENCE OF INDEPENDENCE

The surveillance architecture documented in Chapter 6 targeted community — specifically, the organized community with the political capacity to investigate and resist what was being done to its members. COINTELPRO's operational objective was not merely to surveil but to atomize: to prevent the formation of the organized social trust that makes collective resistance possible.

The inverse of that objective is the specific resilience that the system feared.

**The Amish as documented case study.* The Amish communities of Ohio, Pennsylvania, and Indiana are not presented here as a religious prescription. They are presented as a documented natural experiment in the health outcomes of communities that have maintained systematic independence from the industrial food system, the pharmaceutical system, and the digitally mediated social architecture of the mainstream culture.

Research published in peer-reviewed journals including the *Journal of Allergy and Clinical Immunology* (Stein et al., 2016) and subsequent studies has documented that Amish children have dramatically lower rates of asthma, allergies, and autoimmune conditions compared to matched populations in the surrounding culture. The mechanisms under investigation include microbial diversity from farm exposure, raw milk consumption, reduced antibiotic use, and the reduced processed food consumption that follows from a food system organized around local production and preparation. The Amish studies are not conclusive on mechanism.

They are significant on outcome. Communities that have maintained independence from specific captured systems show systematically different health profiles from communities that have not.

The principle generalizes beyond the Amish. Documented research on traditional food cultures — the Mediterranean dietary patterns studied by Ancel Keys and subsequently in the Lyon Diet Heart Study, the traditional Japanese dietary patterns documented in centenarian research, the documented health profiles of communities with high dietary diversity and low processed food consumption — consistently shows that populations eating food that closely resembles what the species ate before industrial processing show lower rates of the chronic conditions the pharmaceutical model manages.

The practical architecture of local community. The specific community structures that reduce dependence on captured systems are not mysterious. They are the structures that the captured systems compete with and, where possible, undermine: the local church, the neighborhood association, the community garden, the farmers' market, the local food cooperative, the mutual aid network. These structures provide the practical functions — social support, shared resources, collective knowledge, childcare, food access, crisis response — that the surveilled digital infrastructure has partially replaced with monitored, algorithmically curated substitutes.

The person who knows their neighbors — who has established relationships of practical reciprocity with the people who live within walking distance — is a fundamentally different node in the network than the person whose social existence is mediated through platforms that monetize the attention and log the behavior. The network of genuine local community is not surveilled at the level the digital infrastructure is, is not dependent on corporate infrastructure to function, and is not subject to the algorithmic manipulation that the behavioral monitoring architecture enables.

This is not nostalgia. It is a structural observation about the difference between communication and community infrastructure that is owned and controlled by the person using it versus infrastructure that is owned and controlled by the institutions this book has documented. The exit is not from modernity. It is from the specific monitored, captured, algorithmically managed modernity that the surveillance architecture was built to produce.

Financial and digital sovereignty. Chapter 6 documented the surveillance architecture's scale. The exit from population-level financial surveillance is not complete — the captured financial system is the most difficult part of the apparatus to exit without significant practical cost. What the partial exit looks like: using cash for transactions that do not require digital tracking; understanding that every digital financial transaction is a data point in a behavioral profile; maintaining relationships of direct economic exchange with local producers and service providers that do not route through corporate platforms; understanding the documented risks of the Central Bank Digital Currency frameworks being developed by multiple governments, which would make the surveillance of financial behavior structurally total.

These are not paranoid precautions. They are the minimum level of understanding about the infrastructure you are using that the documented record of this book requires. The person who understands what their phone tracks, what their credit card records, what their grocery store loyalty program logs, and what their smart home device transmits is a person making informed choices about the infrastructure they use. That is not a lifestyle prescription. It is the minimum standard of informed consent applied to the digital environment.

IV. THE THEOLOGY OF THE EXIT

This chapter has been, up to this point, a practical document. That is intentional. The exit has practical content. It does not float above the daily decisions of the person who eats, who sees a doctor, who lives in a neighborhood, who uses a phone. It lives in those decisions.

But the practical content is not the reason the exit matters. The reason the exit matters is named in the verse that opens this chapter and in the verse the Introduction quoted on its third page.

Come out of her, my people. The command is not addressed to the politically aware, or to the nutritionally informed, or to the health-conscious, or to the privacy-minded. It is addressed to *my people* — the ones who belong to the one who is speaking. The ones whose bodies are temples of the Holy Spirit, as Paul wrote to the Corinthians. The ones whose biological integrity was assaulted in every program this book documents not because they happened to be accessible but because the one who breathed life into the first human being placed something of infinite value in every human body — and the assault, across a hundred years of documented institutional programs, has been specifically and consistently aimed at that.

The person who grows their own food, who maintains their medical history, who knows their neighbors, who understands the surveillance infrastructure they are using — that person is practicing a form of resistance that the system fears for specific reasons. The system's economic health depends on the managed dependence of the person who does not do these things. Every act of genuine self-sufficiency is a withdrawal from that dependence. Every relationship of local community that does not route through a corporate platform is a node in a network the surveillance architecture cannot fully map. Every patient who exercises informed consent is a patient the protocol cannot automatically process.

These things are worth doing on purely practical grounds. The documentation supports them.

But they are worth doing for a deeper reason that the documentation cannot supply. The body you are caring for, the food you are feeding it, the community you are building around it — these are not your possessions. They were given. The one who gave them is the one holding the rope that has been visible from the first page of this book. The call to come out of the system is inseparable from the call to come to him — not as a political movement, not as a wellness program, not as an identity community, but as the response to the one who said:

I came that they may have life, and have it abundantly.

The abundant life is not a promise about freedom from difficulty. The reader who has followed thirteen chapters of documented assault knows that the people who answered that call before us did not receive exemption from difficulty. What they received was the one thing the apparatus cannot provide and cannot take: the relationship with the one who made them, who holds them, and who is calling them out.

The next chapter is not a chapter of documentation. It is a chapter of call. Chapter 14 ends here, at the threshold. What comes next is the decision.

PRIMARY SOURCES AND RESOURCES FOR THIS CHAPTER

Food Sovereignty and Seed Saving:

- Seed Savers Exchange, seedsavers.org. The largest open-source seed library in the United States, maintaining more than 20,000 varieties of open-pollinated seeds. Membership provides access to seed trading among a community of growers outside the commercial seed system.

- Organic Seed Alliance, seedalliance.org. Research, education, and advocacy organization focused on the preservation and development of open-pollinated seed varieties. Publishes research on seed sovereignty and the documented decline of seed diversity in the commercial system.

- Svalbard Global Seed Vault, seedvault.no. The international backup facility for the world's seed banks, holding more than 1.4 million seed samples. Its existence is itself documentation of what is at stake in the concentration of seed ownership.

The Suppressed Dietary Science:

- Kearns, Cristin E., Laura A. Schmidt, and Stanton A. Glantz, "Sugar Industry and Coronary Heart Disease Research: A Historical Analysis of Internal Industry Documents," *JAMA Internal Medicine* 176(11), November 2016. The landmark paper documenting the Sugar Research Foundation's funding of research designed to shift blame for coronary heart disease from sugar to fat. Available at jamanetwork.com.

- Teicholz, Nina, *The Big Fat Surprise: Why Butter, Meat and Cheese Belong in a Healthy Diet* (Simon & Schuster, 2014). Comprehensive review of the peer-reviewed literature on dietary fat, drawing on primary research studies and documenting the institutional suppression of findings that contradicted the fat-hypothesis consensus.

- Taubes, Gary, *Good Calories, Bad Calories: Fats, Carbs, and the Controversial Science of Diet and Health* (Anchor Books, 2008). The foundational documented account of the science of dietary fat and carbohydrate, tracing the history of the research and the political processes by which dietary guidelines were shaped.

Direct Primary Care:

- Direct Primary Care Alliance, dpcare.org. National membership organization for DPC practices, maintaining a directory of participating physicians searchable by location.

- Garrison, Lisa, et al., "Direct Primary Care: An Innovative Alternative Practice Model," *Journal of the American Board of Family Medicine* 30(5), September-October 2017. Peer-reviewed documentation of the DPC model's structure, outcomes, and evidence base.

- Eskew, Phillip M., and Katherine Klink, "Direct Primary Care: Practice Distribution and Cost Across the Nation," *Journal of the American Board of Family Medicine* 28(6), November-December 2015. Peer-reviewed analysis of DPC's distribution and cost structure.

Informed Consent:

- The Nuremberg Code (1947), available through the U.S. Holocaust Memorial Museum at ushmm.org. The foundational international standard. Ten principles. Readable in five minutes. The reader who has not read it should.

- U.S. Department of Health and Human Services, "The Belmont Report: Ethical Principles and Guidelines for the Protection of Human Subjects of Research" (1979), available at hhs.gov. The American framework for research ethics, adopted in response to the Tuskegee revelation.

- HIPAA Privacy Rule, 45 CFR Part 164. The federal framework governing patient access to their own medical records. Available at hhs.gov. Every patient has the right to a complete copy of their medical record.

Community Resilience Research:

- Stein, Michelle M., et al., "Innate Immunity and Asthma Risk in Amish and Hutterite Farm Children," *New England Journal of Medicine* 375(5), August 4, 2016. The peer-reviewed study documenting dramatically lower asthma rates in Amish children, with analysis of mechanisms related to farm exposure and microbial diversity.

- de Lorgeril, Michel, et al., "Mediterranean Diet, Traditional Risk Factors, and the Rate of Cardiovascular Complications After Myocardial Infarction," *Circulation* 99(6), February 16, 1999. The Lyon Diet Heart Study — the randomized controlled trial of Mediterranean dietary intervention showing 72% reduction in cardiac events. Available at ahajournals.org.

Surveillance and Digital Sovereignty:

- The Intercept, Snowden documents archive — theintercept.com. The primary document archive for the NSA surveillance programs revealed by Snowden. The reader who wants to understand the scope of the behavioral surveillance infrastructure is directed to the documents themselves.

- Electronic Frontier Foundation, eff.org. The primary civil liberties organization documenting digital surveillance infrastructure, maintaining accessible guides to privacy practices organized by threat model. Not advocacy — documented technical analysis.

- Bank for International Settlements, "CBDCs: An Opportunity for the Monetary System," BIS Annual Economic Report 2021, Chapter III — bis.org. The BIS's own documentation of the Central Bank Digital Currency framework, including its implications for financial surveillance. The reader who wants to understand what is being built is directed to the primary documents of the institutions building it.

The resources in this chapter are not hidden. They are available to anyone willing to look. The exit from a captured system does not require extraordinary resources or extraordinary courage. It requires the willingness to act on what the documented record shows — one decision, one habit, one relationship, one garden at a time.

Chapter 15: The Only Hope

The Rope, the Name, and the Call

"The thief comes only to steal and kill and destroy. I came that they may have life and have it abundantly."

— John 10:10

"If you confess with your mouth that Jesus is Lord and believe in your heart that God raised him from the dead, you will be saved."

— Romans 10:9

You have seen it clearly.

Fourteen chapters of documented evidence. Congressional transcripts. FOIA-released documents. Peer-reviewed scientific literature. The published statements of the principals themselves. The eugenics movement's funded ideology and the law it became. The pharmaceutical monopoly built by the same money. The experimental programs — MKUltra, Tuskegee, the radiation experiments — and the institutional culture that made them normal. The suppression architecture designed to neutralize the communities most directly harmed. The regulatory capture. The food system. The childhood vaccine schedule's removed liability. The Epstein enforcement network. The global coordination mechanism. The hospital protocols of 2020. The defense-funded platform technology, the suppressed origins question, the private channels specifically designed to leave no record.

You have not been deceived about what the record shows. The documentation is real. The pattern is real. The assault on the human body and human cognition — across a hundred years, across institutional generations, converging with increasing precision and scale — is real.

This chapter does not add to that record. It does something different. It names what the record has been demanding that we name since the first chapter. And then it extends the only call adequate to what the record demands.

I. THE WORLD AS IT IS

Three texts, speaking across millennia, describing the same thing.

From the Gospel of Luke — the temptation of Jesus, in the wilderness, the enemy showing him all the kingdoms of the world in a moment of time: *"And the devil said to Him, 'All this authority I will give You, and their glory; for this has been delivered to me, and I give it to whomever I wish.'"*

From the letter of John — written at the end of the first century, after the apostle had watched the church take root across the Roman world and had watched the world try to consume it: *"We know that we are of God, and the whole world lies under the sway of the wicked one."*

From the letter of James — to Jewish believers scattered across the empire, practical and blunt and demanding: *"Do you not know that friendship with the world is enmity with God?"*

These three texts land on the same diagnosis. The world as currently ordered is not a neutral environment in which human beings make free choices among equally available options. It is a managed system under the governance of a specific intelligence whose nature — whose operational description, as Jesus gave it — is theft and destruction.

The authority was delivered to him. He said so himself, to Jesus, who did not dispute the claim. What he offered Jesus — all the kingdoms, all their glory — is what he has been distributing ever since to everyone willing to make the trade. The documented history of this book is the institutional record of those trades: the funding, the capture, the managed systems, the suppression of everything that threatens the arrangement.

The evidence assembled in the preceding fourteen chapters is the documentation of that governance in institutional form. The thief does not announce himself. He builds systems. He captures institutions. He funds ideologies. He organizes the incentive structures that produce predictable human behavior without requiring that any individual in the system know whose purposes they are serving. He has been doing this, in documented form, for a hundred years of American institutional history.

II. THE INDICTMENT THAT INCLUDES EVERYONE

The book of Romans says one thing plainly, with a sustained force drawn from the accumulated testimony of the Psalms and the prophets:

There is none righteous, no, not one. There is none who understands; there is none who seeks after God. They have all turned aside; they have together become unprofitable. Their throat is an open tomb; with their tongues they have practiced deceit. Their feet are swift to shed blood; destruction and misery are in their ways; and the way of peace they have not known. There is no fear of God before their eyes.

Paul is not describing the oligarchs. He is not describing the CIA officials who designed MKUltra, or the Public Health Service physicians who watched syphilis kill for forty years, or the researchers who injected plutonium into patients who came for treatment of their cancer. He is describing everyone. He cites the Psalms because the Psalms were written by and about the people of God — the covenant community, the ones with the law and the prophets and the presence of the living God in their midst.

Everyone. Without exception.

The fallen nature that the destroying mind exploits in the oligarchs — the hunger for wealth, for protection, for the intoxicating certainty of being on the winning side — lives in every human being. The reader who has spent fourteen chapters documenting institutional evil is not therefore clean. The capacity for the same trades, under the same pressures, under sufficient incentive and sufficient fear, exists in every person reading this page.

This is not said to minimize what the documented record shows. The specific people who made the specific decisions documented in these chapters bear specific responsibility for what they did. That is real and should not be softened. But the indictment that Romans assembles does not allow the reader to exit the dock through the back door of moral superiority. The pen holds everyone. The rope is for everyone. The rescue is not for the virtuous. It is for the human.

III. THE STORY THE OLD TESTAMENT TELLS

The Old Testament is the story of what God did when the world the first chapters of Genesis describe — the creation breathed into existence, the image-bearers set to tend it, the intimate relationship between Creator and creature — was broken.

He did not abandon it. He called one man: Abraham, from Ur of the Chaldees, with no credentials and no reason given except the call itself. From that man a family. From that family a people. From that people a covenant — *I will be your God, and you shall be my people* — carved into stone on a mountain in the desert. From that covenant a law, a temple, a sacrificial system that kept pointing, generation after generation, to a remedy whose full nature the participants could not yet see. From that people, in the fullness of time, the Son of God was born.

The Old Testament is not a record of the people of Israel's virtue. It is a record of God's faithfulness in the face of their persistent failure to be what they were called to be — and his refusal to abandon the project because the project was never primarily about them. It was about the one who was coming through them. The call was to one man, from one man a people, from that people the Messiah, and through the Messiah an offer extended to every human being who has ever lived.

The Hebrew people remain precious in God's sight. Paul, who wrote the sharpest description of human fallenness in the biblical canon, also wrote: *"I could wish that I myself were accursed and cut off from Christ for the sake of my brothers, my kinsmen according to the flesh."* The promises made to Abraham have not been revoked. But the focus of the new covenant — the one the old covenant was always pointing toward — is the one who fulfilled it, and in whom every human being, from every tribe and tongue and people and nation, is invited to find what Israel's covenant promised and the sacrificial system could only picture.

The new covenant is not a replacement of the old. It is its completion.

IV. THE NAME

The angel said to the shepherds: *"Fear not, for behold, I bring you good news of great joy that will be for all the people. For unto you is born this day in the city of David a Savior, who is Christ the Lord."*

He taught in the synagogues and in the wilderness where people gathered to him. He went from place to place healing the sick, giving sight to the blind, raising the dead. He sent his disciples in pairs to do likewise. The religious leaders — the institutional authorities of his own people, who had built an interpretive tradition so elaborate that the simple gospel was buried beneath it

— watched his authority with a fear that eventually expressed itself as murderous jealousy. The entire twenty-third chapter of Matthew records Jesus's confrontation with them: *"Woe to you, scribes and Pharisees, hypocrites!"* — seven times, the full weight of prophetic condemnation on those who had taken the keys of the kingdom of heaven and neither entered themselves nor allowed those who wanted to enter.

He cleared the temple with a whip, overturning the tables of the money changers. *"My house shall be called a house of prayer, but you have made it a den of thieves."* The institution had been captured. The system that was supposed to mediate the relationship between the people and God had been converted into an instrument of commerce and control. He drove it out.

The parallels to the documented history of this book are not forced. They are structural. The pattern of institutional capture — of systems designed to mediate healing and protection being converted into instruments of managed dependence — is not new. It is as old as the human capacity to build institutions and sell them to the destroying mind.

He was killed for the disruption he caused. The religious leaders who had the most to lose from his authority arranged it. The Roman governor who had the political power to stop it lacked the courage. The crowd that had celebrated his entry into Jerusalem five days earlier demanded his execution. All of this was the mechanism of human fallenness operating exactly as it has always operated, being used by the destroying mind to accomplish what the destroying mind exists to accomplish: the elimination of the one whose presence in the world represented the specific threat that no institutional capture, no surveillance architecture, no suppression program could neutralize.

He was killed.

And then he walked out of death.

This is the claim that either changes everything or changes nothing. There is no middle position. A man who was dead on Friday afternoon and alive on Sunday morning — not resuscitated, not hallucinated, but physically present and recognizable and eating fish on a beach with his friends — is either the most important event in the history of the world or it did not happen.

The apostles who witnessed it went to their deaths — most of them — rather than retract it. Thomas, who had refused to believe until he put his hand in the wounds, went to India. Andrew went to what is now Georgia and Ukraine. Peter went to Rome. Paul, who had been present at the stoning of Stephen and had hunted the early believers across the Roman world, was personally confronted by the risen Christ on the road to Damascus and spent the rest of his life building the church he had been destroying — and was beheaded in Rome, in the same city where Peter was crucified upside down.

Men do not die for what they know to be a lie. They die for what they believe to be true, and they recant when the cost of belief becomes too high. None of the apostles recanted. John, the one who lived to old age, wrote from exile on Patmos a document that the church has been reading and arguing about ever since.

V. THE RESCUE AND WHAT IT IS

The roadmap for this chapter includes a passage from the Revelation of John that lands with a force that no paraphrase can carry, so it is placed here in its own words:

"And they sang a new song, saying: You are worthy to take the scroll, and to open its seals; for You were slain, and have redeemed us to God by Your blood out of every tribe and tongue and people and nation, and have made us kings and priests to our God; and we shall reign on the earth."

Every tribe. Every tongue. Every people. Every nation.

The rescue is not ethnic. It is not cultural. It is not available only to people who were raised in one tradition or who came to it in one way. The blood that purchases the redemption was poured out for everyone the thief came to steal from, kill, and destroy. The offer is open. The terms are not negotiable — they cannot be, because the price has already been paid, and the one who paid it is the only one with the standing to name the terms — but they are available to every person who will receive them.

What is the rescue from?

First and most fundamentally: from the consequence of what every human being is and has done. The indictment Paul assembled from the Psalms and the prophets is not rhetorical. It describes a condition — the condition of the creature separated from its Creator, operating according to its own judgment in a world under the governance of the destroying mind, accumulating the spiritual debt that the law could name but not discharge. The rescue is from that debt, paid in full by the one who had no debt of his own and chose to take the debt of everyone who would receive him.

Second: from the flesh — the orientation toward self, toward appetite, toward the short-term calculation that has made every human being in this book's documented history susceptible to the trades the destroying mind offers. Paul describes it with clinical precision: *"The works of the flesh are evident: adultery, fornication, uncleanness, lewdness, idolatry, sorcery, hatred, contentions, jealousies, outbursts of wrath, selfish ambitions, dissensions, heresies, envy, murders, drunkenness, revelries."* This is not a list of exceptional vices. It is a description of ordinary human nature operating without the Spirit of God. The oligarchs in this book did not become what they became by being monsters.

They became what they became by being human, with ordinary human hungers, in an institutional environment that rewarded those hungers without limit. The flesh they served is the same flesh every reader carries.

The rescue from the flesh is not willpower. It is not discipline or moral resolution or the grim determination to be better. Paul is explicit: *"Walk in the Spirit, and you shall not fulfill the lust of the flesh."* The Spirit is the operative agent. The person who has received the rescue has received the indwelling presence of the Holy Spirit — the same Spirit that raised Jesus from the dead — as a deposit, a guarantee, a down payment on the full restoration that is coming.

Third: from the pen itself. Not immediately, not completely, not without the difficulty that Chapter 14 acknowledged and that this chapter does not minimize. The world still lies under the governance of the wicked one. The apparatus documented in this book is still operating. The reader who has come to faith does not exit into a life of ease and exemption. What they exit into is a life with a different orientation — no longer toward the pen's managed endpoints but toward the one who entered the pen from outside it and who holds the rope.

VI. THE CALL

The blueprint for this chapter specified three imperatives. They are stated plainly.

**Repent.* Not of reading this book. Not of seeing what the documented record shows. Of the sin that the record names without naming: the specific ways in which every reader has, in their own life, made the trades the destroying mind offers — traded integrity for security, truth for belonging, the image of God for the approval of the institution. Repentance is not self-punishment. It is a turning — a literal change of direction, from the orientation toward the pen's managed endpoints to the orientation toward the one who calls.

James describes the texture of genuine repentance with a severity that our therapeutic culture finds uncomfortable: _"Lament and mourn and weep. Let your laughter be turned to mourning and your joy to gloom. Humble yourselves in the sight of the Lord, and He will lift you up."_ The lifting up follows the humbling. The order matters. The rescue is not available to the person who is not aware of needing it.

Turn. To Jesus Christ. Not as a philosophical position. Not as a cultural affiliation. Not as a political alignment or a conspiracy-community identity. As the one who walked out of death, who is alive now, and who made a specific offer: "Come to me, all who labor and are heavy laden, and I will give you rest." _Romans 10:9 states the terms with the simplicity that has always marked the gospel:_ "If you confess with your mouth that Jesus is Lord and believe in your heart that God raised him from the dead, you will be saved." Confess. Believe. That is the door.

What follows the door is a life — the life that Paul describes throughout his letters as walking in the Spirit, putting on the armor of God, crucifying the flesh, running the race that is set before us, working out our salvation with fear and trembling while the one who began the work continues it. It is not an easy life. Every one of the apostles who turned experienced exactly how unclean the life that follows becomes. The armor is not decoration. It is equipment for a war that does not end until the end.

But it is the abundant life. The one that was stolen and that the thief cannot reach in the person who has received the rescue.

Come out. Not only from the food system, the pharmaceutical framework, the surveillance architecture, the captured institutions

— though Chapter 14 documented all of that. From the deeper captivity that those systems exploit: the captivity to fear, to appetite, to the assumption that the world as currently managed is the only world available, that the pen is permanent, that there is no rope.

The rope is real. It has been in the room since the first sentence of this book. The hand holding the other end has been holding it through every chapter — through every program, every capture, every stolen life documented in these pages — without letting go.

VII. THE OVERCOMERS

The Revelation of Jesus Christ contains messages to seven churches, and in each message a specific promise to the one who overcomes. The promises are staggering in their scope — to eat from the tree of life in the paradise of God; to be unharmed by the second death; to receive hidden manna and a white stone with a new name; to have authority over the nations; to be clothed in white with your name remaining in the Book of Life; to be made a pillar in the temple, inscribed with the name of God and the name of the new Jerusalem; to sit with Christ on his throne.

These are not rewards for exceptional virtue. They are the inheritance of everyone who overcomes.

Overcomes what?

John answers his own question in the letters: *"I write to you, young men, because you have overcome the wicked one."* And: *"For whatever is born of God overcomes the world. And this is the victory that has overcome the world — our faith."* And the voice from heaven in Revelation 12, after the dragon is cast down: *"And they overcame him by the blood of the Lamb and by the word of their testimony, and they did not love their lives to the death."*

The blood of the Lamb — the rescue, received. The word of their testimony — the witness, given. Not loving their lives to the death — the orientation toward what is coming rather than toward what is being lost.

This is the position of the person who has received what this chapter describes. Not above the war. Not exempt from the difficulty. Not promised ease or comfort or protection from the apparatus documented in thirteen chapters of this book. But positioned — inside the rescue, holding the rope, bearing the testimony — as the one who has already, in the most fundamental sense, won.

The war in Revelation 12 that precedes the dragon's casting down ends with an observation that should land with full force on the reader who has followed this book from its first page: *"Therefore rejoice, O heavens and you who dwell in them! But woe to you, O earth and sea, for the devil has come down to you in great wrath, because he knows that his time is short."*

The apparatus documented in this book is not evidence of the enemy's strength. It is evidence of his desperation. The time is short. He knows it. The escalating assault on the human body and human cognition — culminating in the global-scale demonstration of 2020 and the brain-computer interface programs now in clinical trials — is not the behavior of a power that is winning. It is the behavior of a power that has read the last chapter and is spending everything he has in the time that remains.

The reader who understands this is not terrified by what the documented record shows. They are sobered by it, and they are resolved.

VIII. THE PEN, ONE MORE TIME

The world you live in is the same world the Introduction described.

The food that is supposed to nourish you has been engineered, through mechanisms documented in Chapter 8, to produce the chronic illness the pharmaceutical system then manages. The medicine that is supposed to heal you operates within a system whose economic health depends on your continued dependence. The agencies built to protect you have been captured by the industries they were supposed to regulate. The information environment you inhabit has been shaped, through the mechanisms documented in every chapter of this book, to make the pen feel like the only available world.

None of that has changed.

What has changed — for the reader who has arrived at this page having received what this chapter describes — is orientation. You are not in the pen the way the pen was designed to contain you. You know what it is. You know whose it is. You know what it is for. And you know that the one who entered it from outside, who was not contained by it even in death, is the one who has been holding the rope from the first page — and who is still holding it now.

The rope is in your hand.

You know whose hand is holding the other end.

What you do next is between you and him.

A note on what follows this book: PHARMED documents the theft and names the rescuer. The third book in this trilogy addresses what the rescuer warned was coming — the most sophisticated assault in the enemy's long campaign, timed for the moment when the world is most desperate to receive it and least equipped to evaluate it clearly.

The assault on the body was preparation. The assault on the soul is the culmination. The strong delusion Paul described in 2 Thessalonians 2 is not a distant theological abstraction. It is being assembled now — in the interfaith architecture, the global governance superstructure, the hidden networks embedded in the institutions of western civilization — and it will arrive with all power, signs, and lying wonders, dressed as the healing of the oldest wounds in human history.

DELUSION equips the reader to recognize the offer when it arrives, to test it against the only criteria sufficient to expose it, and to hold the love of the truth at the cost the holding will require. It also names what the overcomer is holding — the seven promises to those who endure, the marriage supper of the Lamb, the genuine resolution of everything the offer will counterfeit.

The rescue named in this chapter is real. What is coming will attempt to replace it with something that wears its face. The third book is about the difference — and about the one who overcomes.

For the reader who cannot wait: the New Testament is available everywhere, in more translations than any document in human history, at no cost. Start with the Gospel of John. Read it in one sitting if you can. The one who wrote it is there.